AF671908

Cardiovascular Aspects of Dialysis Treatment

Cardiovascular Aspects of Dialysis Treatment

The importance of volume control

By

Evert J Dorhout Mees

SPRINGER-SCIENCE+BUSINESS MEDIA, B.V.

A C.I.P. Catalogue record for this book is available from the Library of Congress

ISBN 978-90-481-5442-5 ISBN 978-94-017-0973-6 (eBook)
DOI 10.1007/978-94-017-0973-6

All Rights Reserved
© 2000 Springer Science+Business Media Dordrecht
Originally published by Kluwer Academic Publishers in 2000
No part of the material protected by this copyright notice may be reproduced or utilized in any form or by any means, electronic or mechanical, including photocopying, recording or by any information storage and retrieval system, without written permission from the copyright owner.

Dedication

To my wife Mia, who supported, criticized and encouraged me throughout my professional life and took a major share in the writing of this book.

Table of Contents

Foreword

I have just re-read the last chapter of this excellent book, which may well become a kind of bible guiding us toward the optimal care of the chronic dialysis patient. Furthermore, writing this foreword provides me with the opportunity of putting into words something that I have wanted to articulate for a long time but never quite got it right.

MDs who are destined to care for chronic dialysis patients should receive special training in the care of chronic disease. A Nephrology fellowship seldom if ever provides any training in this discipline. Furthermore, young physicians who choose Nephrology usually are not interested in the chronically ill. Yet, as clearly pointed out in this book, physicians caring for dialysis patients need the same dedication and the same skills that are required for those who are willing to care for other chronic illnesses.

This volume describes in a clear concise manner the critical knowledge needed to achieve and maintain life-preserving normotension in the dialysis patient. However, application of this knowledge to successfully control blood pressure in the dialysis patient demands that sufficient time and careful attention be paid to each individual patient's continually changing fluid balance status. Dry weight, and the normal blood pressure that goes with it, is a constantly changing value that must be re-determined with each dialysis. Since it is easier to give a pill and pretend that one is treating hypertension in the dialysis patient, hypertension is so poorly controlled worldwide that an epidemic of its numerous complications is now present in the world's dialysis population.

One hopes that, with this book now available, this epidemic will gradually be reversed in the decades ahead.

Belding H. Scribner
Seattle, Washington
January 2000

Preface

Many excellent textbooks on chronic dialysis treatment exist, concise as well as comprehensive. Why then yet another book, and one that addresses only part of the problems encountered during this treatment?

Cardiovascular complications not only are responsible for more than half of our patients' mortality, they also represent the bulk of everyday problems in a dialysis unit. Yet the space allotted to them in the textbooks covers only 2–8% of their total content. Moreover they are often not presented in such a way that the treating physician and nurse can easily apply this knowledge to the individual patient. This is one of the reasons why overall results of dialysis treatment have not improved as they could have, despite increasingly more sophisticated machines, biocompatible membranes and formulae to calculate "adequacy of dialysis".

The plan to write this book originated during the 8 years that I had the opportunity to work at the Ege University in Izmir, Turkey. For the second time in my career I engaged in the daily care of dialysis patients. It gradually became clear that systematic application of well-known pathophysiological principles could improve their condition even beyond my expectations. More importantly, it appeared that world literature was concerned mainly with evaluating risk factors and that efforts to improve prognosis were concentrated on urea removal. It is symptomatic that "volume control", which will be the central issue of this book, is not incorporated into the "adequacy" concept.

Some experienced nephrologists have warned against the negligence of these principles, but their voices are like "calling in the desert" of modern technological, commercialized medicine. The implication of these simple concepts has been proven difficult in practice (fig. 1). Both patients and treating staff may become discouraged when instant success is not apparent. As a result, publications casting doubt on "old truths" and suggesting new "factors" have prevailed during recent years. This inevitably creates a bias by mass effect. It is the aim of this book to restore the balance.

Once on dialysis, the patient will not die from "uremia", as used to be his fate before the advent of this treatment. Consequently, the dialysis doctor needs not be a nephrologist. He becomes a "meta-nephrologist"[1] and should specialize in circulatory and cardiac pathophysiology. However, the

---

[1]This term was first used by Dr. Jan Brod in 1969 quoted by Shaldon (ref. 6 Chapter 2)

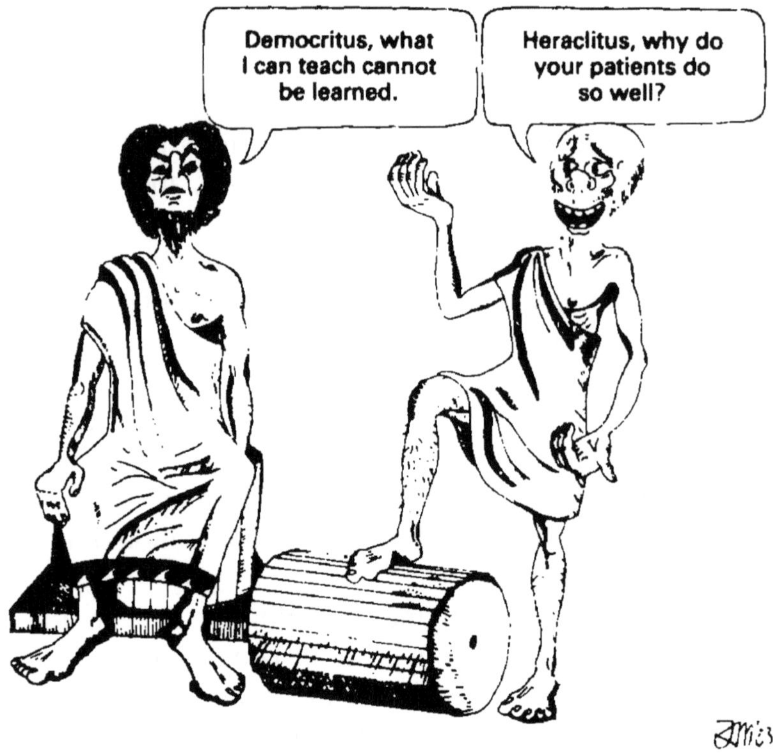
Democritus, what
I can teach cannot
be learned.
Heraclitus, why do
your patients do
so well?

Figure 1 The problem that presents itself to all debutant metanephrologists. From Shaldon and Koch (1985) with permission (ref Ch. 2).

events leading to cardiac problems are quite different from these, which the cardiologist usually encounters.

While the purpose of this book is to give advice which is directly applicable, it is my conviction that an understanding of the physiological background is indispensable. Thus the first chapter deals with some well-known physiological principles, as experience shows that some misconceptions start here. Then the pathophysiological results of salt and volume retention leading to cardiac disease and death are described, as systematically as possible, in the following chapters. However, it has been necessary to discuss on several occasions the most important but complicated relationships between volume and blood pressure and the effects of dialysis upon it.

All other factors, well known as well as speculative, will be mentioned only briefly. I do not intend to deny their potential importance, but modifying them has not (yet) been shown to feasible in practice.

A selected list of references is given at the end of each chapter in alphabetical order. As the titles are mostly self-explanatory, they will be specifically referred to in the text only occasionally.

In dialysis treatment, teamwork is indispensable. All the members of this team, which includes doctor, nurse, patient, often a dietician and family members, should be familiar with the simple rules of "salt and water". While this book is intended mainly for dialysis doctors, I sincerely hope that dialysis nurses will also read it. After all, they are the ones who do nearly all the work and carry (willingly or not) a great responsibility.

Acknowledgements

I am indebted to the patients, doctors and nurses of the Nephrological Department of the Ege University, Izmir, Turkey, for their readiness to help which enabled me to gain invaluable new experience.

My thanks go to Prof. Dr. Ilhan Vidinel for inviting me to work there and to Prof. Dr. Ali Bascı, Prof. Dr. Gürhun Atabay and Doc. Dr. Fehmi Akcicek who gave me support and helpful information in their department.

The remarkable team of friends and colleagues with whom I worked in daily cooperation consisting of Dr. Mustafa Cirit, Doc. Dr. Ercan Ok, Dr. Mehmet Özkahya, Dr. Hüseyin Töz, Doc. Dr. Abdulkadir Ünsal, and many others, were responsible for most of the results upon which this book is based.

Special thanks go to Dr. Branko Braam for critically reviewing the manuscript.

Abbreviations

BP	blood pressure
BV	blood volume
CAPD	continuous ambulatory peritoneal dialysis
CEI	converting enzyme inhibitor
CHF	congestive heart failure
Cti	cardiothoracic index
CV	cardiovascular
DH	dialysis hypotension
ECV	extracellular volume
EF	ejection fraction (of left ventricle)
EPO	erythropoietin
ESRD	end-stage renal disease
HD	hemodialysis
Ht	hematocrit
LVH	left ventricular hypertrophy
MR	mitral regurgitation
PRA	plasma renin activity
TR	tricuspid regurgitation
UF	ultrafiltration

1

Normal physiology

WATER, SALT AND BODY FLUID VOLUMES

Normal values

The body of a normal adult consists for 65% of water. The greater part of this is *intracellular* fluid, the rest *extracellular* fluid. A separate compartment is the *blood volume* (BV), which comprises erythrocytes (red blood cells) and plasma. The proportion of the blood taken up by erythrocytes is called hematocrit.

A healthy non-obese man of 70 kg has approximately[1] an intracellular volume (ICV) of 28 L, an extracellular volume (ECV) of 17 L, a plasma volume of 3 L and an erythrocyte volume of 2 L: and as a consequence a hematocrit of 0.40 (40%) (Figure 1.1). If we subtract the plasma volume from the ECV, the resulting volume represents the *interstitial volume*, which is in this case 14 L. We should realize that if a patient is anemic (as often occurs in terminal renal failure) his 'normal' plasma volume at a hematocrit of 20% is 4 L and his ECV 18 L.

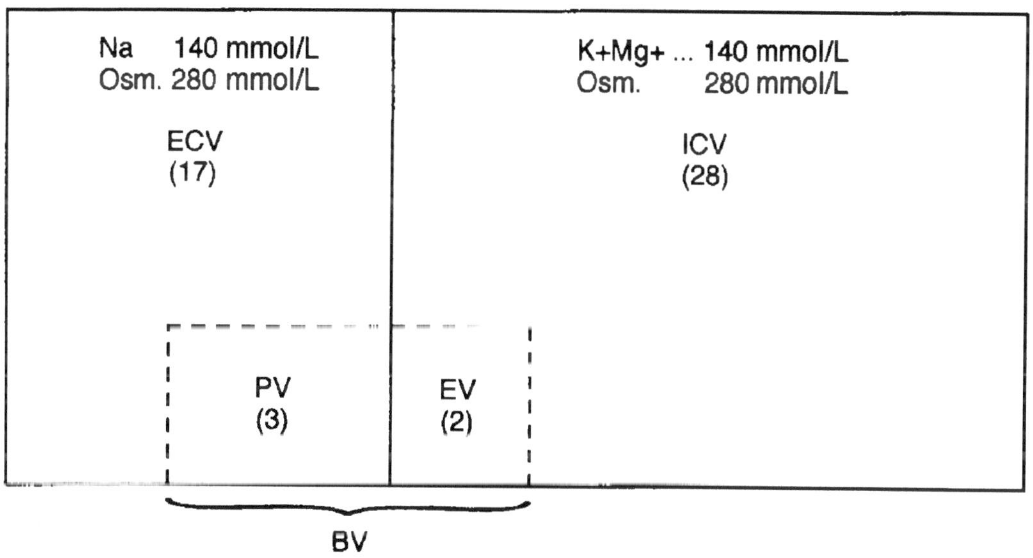

Figure 1.1 Schematic presentation of body fluid compartments. Abbreviations: see text.

[1] These values depend on the methods used. Some authors give lower values for ECV and higher for ICV.

Rules of distribution

The cell membranes, which separate intracellular volume (ICV) from ECV, are freely permeable to water. How do these compartments keep their normal relationship? The answer is that they are impermeable to 'osmotic solutes'. Despite a completely different composition of their solutes, the osmolality[2] of intra- and extracellular fluid is always the same. Thus their 'water content' (which is the reverse of osmolality) is also the same. This is the first 'rule of the body fluids'. Because water can pass through the membranes it is equally distributed over all compartments. Any change in *extracellular* osmolality will immediately be followed by a similar change in *intracellular* osmolality. Thus if pure water is added to the ECV, more than half of it will go to the ICV because this is larger. Conversely, water withdrawal will mainly cause decrease of the ICV. This is one of the reasons why water restriction is relatively ineffective in decreasing the ECV. Similarly, adding salt to the ECV will (apart from causing thirst) increase the ECV by attracting water from the cells. Examples are given in Figure 1.2.

Although a very large number of different molecules are present in the ECV (and plasma) the only quantitatively important solute is the Na-ion and its accompaning anions (Cl- and HCO). As the sum of the latter (because of electric equilibrium) is always equal to Na, we can for all practical purposes estimate the osmolality of plasma by determining the sodium concentration. Indeed the normal osmolality 280 m osm/l, exactly twice the normal Na concentration (140 m osm/L). The reason that all the other solutes (including K, Ca, glucose, etc.) do not seem to contribute is that 'effective osmotic activity' is less than the calculated amount of particles according to van 't Hoffs law.

Because the 'osmoregulation' is kept very strictly, the extracellular volume is usually equivalent to total body Na: ECV (liter) = total body sodium/140. This is the second 'rule of body fluids'. Accordingly, when the ECV is expanded, large excesses in Na are also present. Determination of Na concentration in the blood does not give information on the Na content of the body. In fact, decreased Na concentration is often accompanied by hypervolemia. If one tries to correct hyponatremia by adding a hypertonic (NaCl) solution, this will mainly serve to increase the ECV further, as shown in the example of Figure 1.2d.

In contrast, *blood sodium concentration* is a reliable estimate of cellular hydration (third 'rule of body fluids'). When the Na level changes, body weight changes are no longer reliable estimates of ECV changes, because they are accompanied by a relatively large shift of water to or from the

---

[2] The term 'osmolarity' indicates the number of osmotic particles in a liter of the solution, while 'osmolality' is that number expressed per kg of water. Because blood serum and plasma contain +7% (lipo) proteins there is a 7% difference between these two measures.

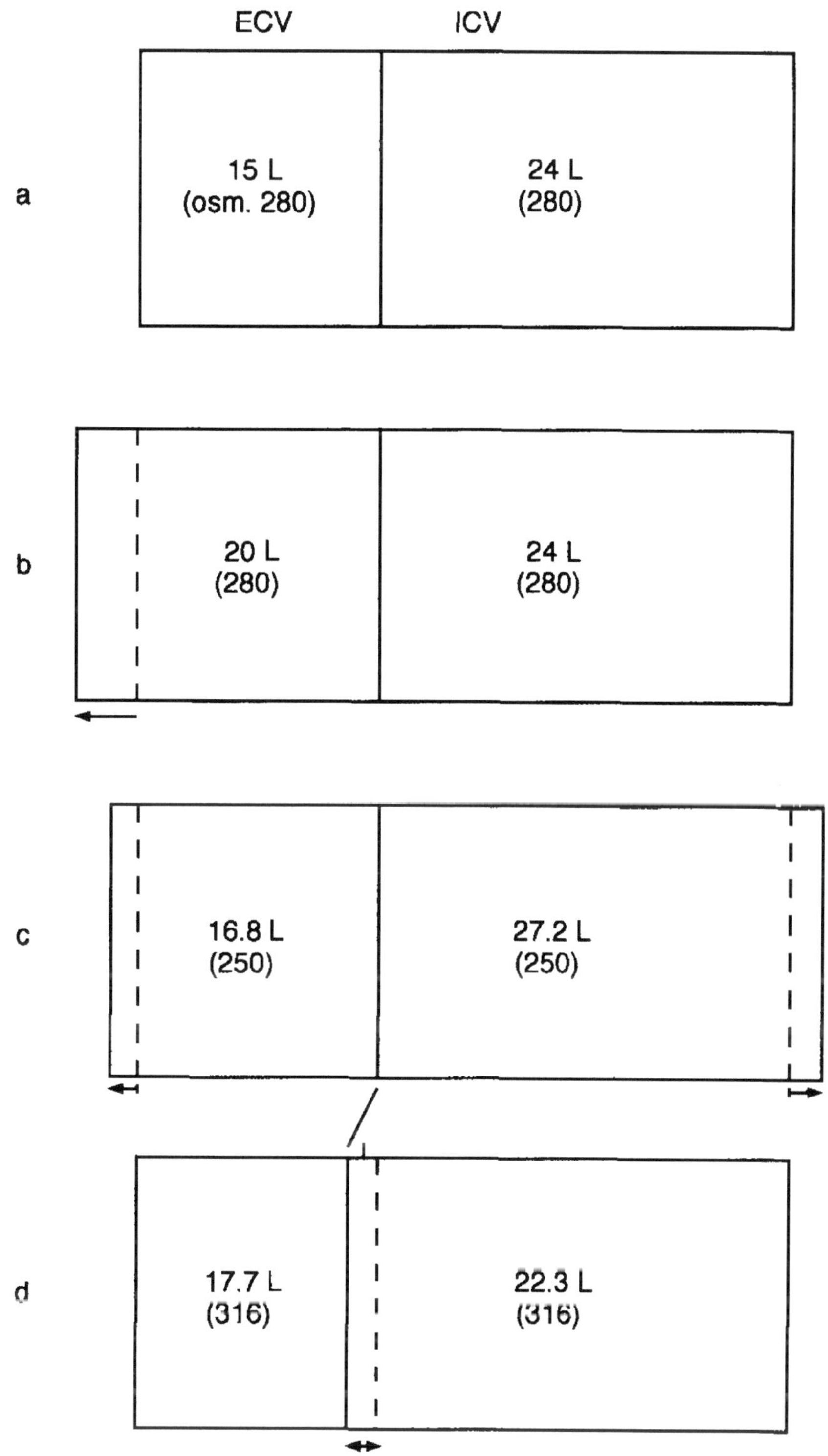

Figure 1.2 Changes in ECV and ICV in a hypothetical subject. Osmolality in brackets. (a) normal condition; (b) addition of 5 L isotonic saline (1400 m mol Na + Cl); (c) addition of 5 L water; (d) addition of 1400 m mol (Na + Cl) without water.

cells. For example, a 10% decrease in Na concentration in a 'standard person' means an excess of 2.6 L (kg) of *intracellular* water.

Although we know the amount of particles in the intracellular fluid (which is the same as in the ECV) its *composition* is completely different (the main cautions being K and Mg) but cannot be measured in clinical practice. However, we may safely assume that their total amount does not change acutely.

Pathological conditions affecting fluid distribution

Urea is a small molecule that, like water, easily crosses the cell membranes. Thus the urea concentration in the cells follows urea concentration in the blood. This means that urea is 'osmotically not active'. In uremic patients osmolality as determined by the freezing-point method will be elevated and should be corrected by subtracting the urea level (60 mg urea = 1 m mol) from the measured value to know 'effective' osmolality. However, when the urea level is rapidly lowered during dialysis, urea diffusion out of the cells lags behind and becomes temporary osmotically active, causing a dysequilibrium (see Chapter 6).

Glucose is osmotically active when elevated (diabetic patients), and will attract fluid from the cells, thus 'diluting' the EC fluid. For instance a glucose level of 35 m mol/l (30 m mol above normal) will increase the ECV by 10% and decrease Na level to the same extent. After normalization the reverse process takes place.

Intoxications with small molecular substances like *alcohol* and *ethylenglycol* (anti-freeze) will also cause measurable increases in blood osmolality. Alcohol, like urea, crosses the cell membranes and is not osmotically active. In fact it increases water excretion by inhibiting anti-diuretic hormone secretion.

How are volumes measured?

Volumes can be determined by injecting a biologically inactive substance, which is known to be distributed only in that compartment and can be measured accurately (usually a radioactive isotope with a short half-life). Dividing the injected amount by the concentration reached after equilibration gives the *distribution volume*. Such *dilution methods* are rather impracticable and have several sources of error, the main being the difficulty to establish the normal value for a certain individual. Therefore in clinical practice, excess or deficit are better estimated on clinical grounds, while acute changes (which are often more interesting than absolute figures) can be accurately *assessed* by *changes* in body weight (for ECV), Na concentration (for ICV) or hematocrit (for BV).

2 REGULATING MECHANISMS IN NORMAL MAN

Osmoregulation

Keeping the extracellular osmolality (Na concentration) constant indirectly controls the intracellular volume, which is of paramount importance for cell function. This is accomplished by two separate mechanisms.

The *first* is the ability of the *kidney* to produce hypertonic urine (3–4 × plasma osmolality) or hypotonic urine (1/5 of plasma osmolality) when hyper- or hypo-osmolality occurs. This osmoregulation works with amazing precision and rapidity. It is so efficient that it is virtually impossible to cause water intoxication in a person with normal kidneys. If a normal person drinks 1 L of water (less than 0.5% of TBW) the kidney, in less than a few hours, excretes this amount. The effector of this regulation, the antidiuretic hormone (ADH or vasopressin), is a polypeptide secreted by the posterior hypophysis, which forces the kidney to produce concentrated urine. When it is suppressed, urine becomes hypo-osmolar.

The second mechanism is *thirst*, which protects against hyperosmolality. This is such a strong urge that hyperosmolality almost never occurs unless the patient is unconscious or is not allowed to drink. The opposite-dislike of drinking as a protection against water intoxication – does not exist, because the kidney, as we have seen, provides enough protection. Also if not under social obligation to drink tea, beer etc. people drink just enough to produce a moderately concentrated urine (particularly in summer) because ADH secretion threshold is below the thirst threshold.

It is evident, however, that with declining renal function, the ability to excrete a water load decreases in parallel, and becomes abolished when end-stage failure occurs. Thus the advice to renal patients, sometimes erroneously given, to drink a large amount of water 'to protect the kidney' or 'to wash away toxic metabolites' lacks a pathophysiological basis and may be harmful. The origin of this widespread belief is that with normal kidneys the clearance of urea is dependent on urine flow, but only at flow rates below 1 ml/min. This is due to urea back-diffusion in the distal nephron from the concentrated filtrate. In patients with decreased renal function this phenomenon does not occur because concentrating power is lost and such low flow rates cannot be achieved any more. As a consequence, their minimal urine volume is higher, as is minimal fluid intake. On the other hand their diluting capacity also becomes impaired, and consequently the maximal water intake that can be excreted is diminished. Thus forced high water consumption may lead to hyponatremia.

In general, *solute exretion* by either the normal or the diseased kidney is *independent of water excretion*, while adequate water intake is safeguarded by the thirst feeling: the body knows better than the doctor. We will come back to other misconceptions in discussions on overhydration.

Regulation of extracellular volume

The ECV completely depends on salt (NaCl) balance. As 'natural' food contains little salt, the mammalian kidney is conditioned to preserve it. In normal conditions the volume of the EC fluid is determined by the total amount of Na in the body, because 'water follows sodium'. When the volume is too low, the kidney can do no more than prevent further loss. There is not such a thing as 'salt hunger'.

Because a 'normal diet' contains more salt than is needed to replace the minute losses by sweat and stools, modern man is constantly threatened by (extracellular) overhydration. The kidneys are thus constantly excreting the excess ingested with the food.

The ability of the kidney to excrete salt is limited. Although its upper limit has never been systematically investigated, available evidence suggests that manifest overhydration (dependent on the individual) will occur when the amount to be excreted is more than 5% of the 'filtered load'. While this still seems a large amount (35 g per day) it should be realized that, when the kidney function of a patient drops below 20% of normal, 5% of it represents more than the salt content of a normal diet.

The way in which the body regulates ECV is one of the unresolved riddles of physiology. A 'volume center' has not been identified. However, it is clear that the mechanisms by which the kidney is informed (afferent pathway) are mediated by changes in *blood volume*, which normally changes in proportion to ECV (Chapter 2). The *efferent pathway* is sodium excretion by the kidney. An important mechanism is 'pressure natriuresis'. In the isolated kidney, salt excretion is directly dependent on blood pressure. In the intact organism, this phenomenon is often not directly apparent, because of many other mechanisms that regulate in an integrated way the vitally important volume homeostasis. Among these the *renin–angiotensin–aldosterone system* (RAAS) is the most important one. This is activated when hypovolemia threatens and is inhibited by hypervolemia.

Angiotensin II has a powerful vasoconstrictive and blood-pressure elevating effect and at the same time stimulates sodium retention by the kidney. Aldosterone also forces the kidney to reabsorb sodium and thus increases ECV and blood volume, which indirectly raises blood pressure (see Chapter 4). According to Guyton (1972), an upward shift of the set point for pressure natriuresis is the basic disturbance causing hypertension. Despite the fact that abnormalities of the RAAS play an important role in different forms of hypertension, phylogenetically this system seems to be primarily related to both salt and volume homeostasis. This is an important issue because, as will be discussed in the next chapters, in dialysis patients normal blood pressure can be achieved in the large majority by manipulating their volume state. Indeed normotension can be associated with a broad range of renin–angiotensin levels. However, hypervolemia almost invariably leads to hypertension, even in the absence of renin.

The *sensitivity* of the volume (salt) regulation is much less than that of osmoregulation. Roughly speaking an increase of 1–1.5 L (8%) is needed to keep the required balance, as shown by the fact that a normal person loses 1–1.5 kg when put on a salt-free diet. Which of the two volumes should be considered as 'normal' and how the 'set point' is determined are interesting questions, but will not be discussed here. The speed of the volume feedback regulation is also much slower than that of osmoregulation: more than 24 hours.

Thus body fluid volumes are controlled by a perfect interaction of osmo regulation and volume regulation. Because the former is more rapid and sensitive, it takes priority in conditions of 'conflict of interest' as stated by John Peters more than 50 years ago. The seeming paradox 'Sodium concentration (osmolality) is determined by water balance, and volume regulation by salt balance, has extremely important clinical consequences. We will come back to this issue in the following chapters.

Summary

- Rules of body fluids:
  1. Osmolality (water content) of ECV and ICV are always equal.
  2. ECV is determined by the total amount of body sodium.
  3. Na concentration is an estimate of cellular hydration.
- *Osmolality* is regulated by the kidney, which can produce urine containing more or less water than the body fluids. However, the thirst mechanism is also able to keep a normal osmolality in the absence of kidney function.
- *Volume regulation* is solely dependent on the sodium excretion by the kidney, which is influenced by an integrated regulatory system in which blood pressure and renin–angiotensin–aldostorone play the most important roles.

Bibliography

Guyton AC, Coleman TG, Cowley AW *et al.* Arterial pressure regulation. Am J Med. 1972;52:584–94.

Peters JP. The role of sodium in the production of edema. New Eng J Med. 1948;239:352.

[3] The antidiuretic hormone (ADH) normally serves osmoregulation and has no function in volume regulation. With extreme hypovolemia it may be activated, but the volume threshold is much higher than the osmotic threshold. This volume stimulus is believed to be mediated by high angiotensin levels.

2

Terminal renal failure

1 THE AIM OF DIALYSIS TREATMENT

As kidney disease progresses, the various renal functions become compromised, until end-stage renal disease (ESRD) occurs, when they are nearly completely lost. While the term ESRD originally implied that the patient could not survive without 'renal replacement' therapy, there is a general tendency to start treatment earlier, while there is still some 'residual' renal function present.

The functions of the kidney may be categorized as follows: 1. Excretion of potentially toxic metabolites; 2. Volume- and osmo-regulation; 3. Hormonal functions: erythropoietin, 1.25 dihydroxycholecalciferol, renin. Dialysis treatment can compensate (1) by dialysis proper and (2) by ultrafiltration, which is usually applied during dialysis, but can also be performed in isolation. Hormonal functions (3) cannot be taken over by dialysis and necessitate administrations of drugs.

Because the most intensive dialysis programs provide not more than 15% of normal kidney function and do this (in the case of hemodialysis) intermittently, some dietary restrictions are logical. Everything which is ingested has to be removed by dialysis. It cannot be stressed enough that the treatment of the patient with ESRD should be *comprehensive* and that dialysis should be integrated within the framework of complete medical, psychological and social care. Experience has shown that the fascination of sophisticated machinery may detract attention from the other aspects of patient care.

For successful dialysis, it is essential that some basic principles are understood not only by the doctor, the dialysis nurses, the dieticians and the social workers, but first of all by the patient himself/herself. To ensure this, repeated talks with the patient, supplemented by written explanations, are necessary. As wrong habits are easily adopted and hard to break, such instructions should be given at an early stage.

Because this book concerns mainly cardiovascular aspects, we will concentrate on the second renal function and its replacement: *volume control,* which is not only the most important, but also the most difficult, and is therefore often neglected. This becomes apparent in the publications on *adequate dialysis,* a subject that merits more detailed discussion.

2 WHEN IS DIALYSIS ADEQUATE?

When the euphoria of the first years after introduction of dialysis treatment was over, it became evident that mortality remained unacceptably high (Figure 2.1). Moreover, the large differences in treatment outcome between centers and countries strongly suggested that these were related to the *way of treatment*. For example, the survival on hemodialysis was, when corrected for age and other illnesses, nearly twice as long in Japan as in the USA (Figure 2.2). This led to the conviction that dialysis, as it is generally practiced, is not adequate.

In 1975 the National Institutes of Health decided to start a National Cooperative Dialysis Study to investigate this problem. This resulted in the concept of *urea kinetic modeling* which showed that not only insufficient dialysis, but also low urea levels due to inadequate nutrition and low *protein catabolic rate*, were associated with increased mortality (Lowrie et al. 1981). Subsequent analysis (Gotch and Sargent 1985) suggested that the effectiveness of treatment should be expressed in the *KT/V* formula: In this concept, *K* is the dialysance of the apparatus, *T* the treatment time (hours per week) and *V* the volume of body fluids (often substituted by body weight). Residual kidney urea clearance can be added. In short, the formula represents total urea clearance standardized by body mass.

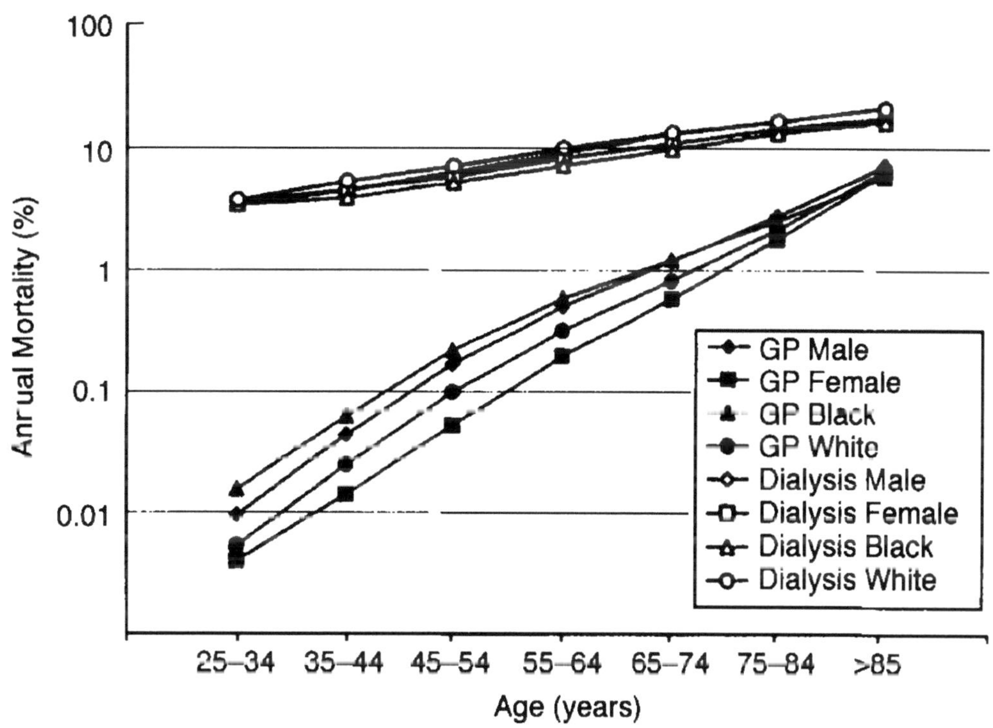

Figure 2.1 Cardiovascular mortality in the general population (Nat Center Health Stat. 1993) and in dialysis patients (U.S. Renal Data Syst 1994–96). Note logarithmic scale. From Levey and Eknoyan 1999, with permission.

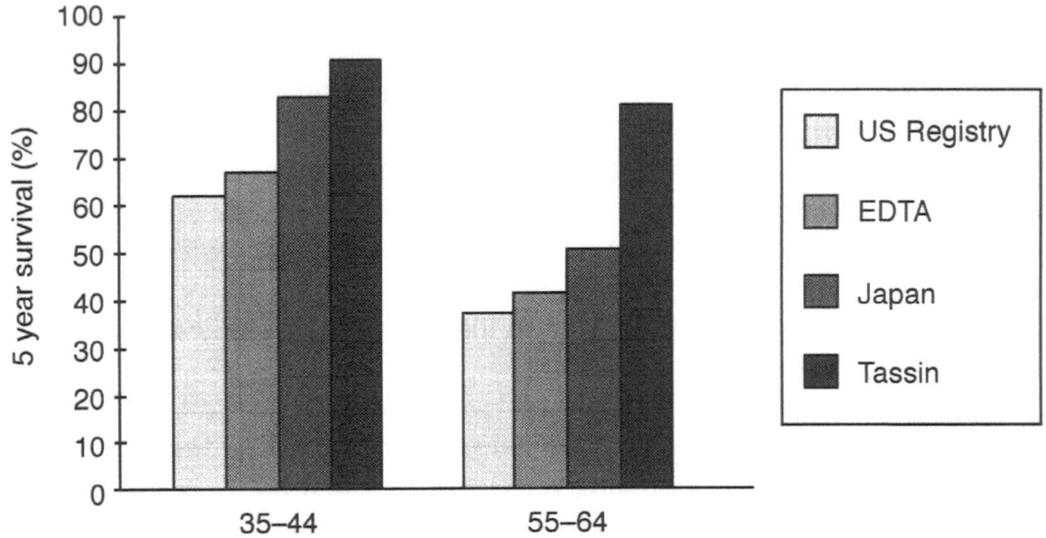

Figure 2.2 Survival rates of dialysis patients age 35–44 and age 55–64 years in different regions in the world and in one center (Tassin, France). Adapted from Charra et al. 1992.

It is amazing how this logical, simple concept conquered the dialysis world as if it were a new evangelic. While it had some favorable effects, it soon appeared to have serious drawbacks. As remarked by Shaldon and Koch (1985) the mechanistic analysis implied with *KT/V* 'being only an appendix to overall assessment of dialysis adequacy, has been promoted to a rigorous statistical tool, further detracting the physician's attention from sound clinical judgement'.

3 CRITICISM OF THE *KT/V* CONCEPT

This concept is based on the premise that urea is an adequate substitute for uremic toxicity, but this is only partly correct. It gives no information on some other aspects of renal failure such as acidosis, anemia and osteodystrophy. A much more serious shortcoming is, however, the implicit assumption that accumulation of toxic substances is the only reason for the dialysis patient's morbidity and that dialysis is adequate when this danger can be diverted. Thus substitution of the kidney's other main task: the regulation of body fluids, circulation and blood pressure is not included. Yet the main cause of morbidity and death is cardiovascular complications, and there is every reason to believe that they are closely related to insufficient correction of these circulatory disturbances, although even this statement is being questioned. The *KT/V* index does not estimate whether or not this most important kidney function has been sufficiently replaced. Thus, this very limited approach, in which dialysis is considered as a drug of which we only have to know the 'dose' which should be 'administered', has led to an inadequate 'adequacy' concept.

One of the results of preoccupation with urea removal was that it stimulated the tendency towards shortening dialysis time, which had started earlier for socio-economic reasons. The use of more permeable ('high-flux') membranes made it possible to achieve a high *KT/V* within a shorter time. The fashion for short dialysis, which started in the USA, was rapidly adopted by the rest of the world. In the UK, for instance, the percentage of patients getting less than 11 hours dialysis a week increased from 25% in 1985 to 42% in 1991. While this did not seem to harm the patients at first sight, long-term effects of short dialysis proved to be deleterious and resulted in increased morbidity and mortality. Such a policy made volume control difficult or impossible, and resulted in the use of more cardiovascular medication and an increased number of episodes with cardiac congestion (Wizemann and Kramer 1987).

Why even a small amount of overhydration is indeed harmful will become clear when we discuss its consequences in the following chapters. First let us see how it happens and how it can be prevented.

4 CONTROL OF ECV IN DIALYSIS PATIENTS

It may be said without exaggeration that nearly all patients with terminal renal failure are overhydrated at the start of dialysis, because their salt intake, even when restricted, exceeds the excretion capacity. Detection of extracellular volume (ECV) excess is not easy and up to 5 L can be retained without evident clinical signs such as edema. One of the great advantages of dialysis treatment is that it enables us to remove this fluid excess, but this has to be repeated during every session because every bit of salt ingested with the diet will cause expansion of the ECV.

Ultrafiltration

There are two methods of removing fluid. We can increase the *osmotic* or the *hydrostatic* gradient between the blood and the dialysis fluid. The first, osmotic ultrafiltration (UF), is used in peritoneal dialysis where a solute (glucose) which does not pass quickly through the peritoneal membrane is added to the rinsing fluid (see Chapter 13). The second, hydrostatic ultrafiltration, can be done by raising the hydrostatic pressure in the blood compartment of the dialyser by putting a clamp on the outflow or by causing negative pressure in the dialysate compartment. In modern machines the latter method is used. UF is usually performed during dialysis. It is, however, better tolerated when applied 'in isolation', without circulating the rinsing fluid. A simple ultrafiltrator consisting of a blood pump and a manometer can be easily constructed. The ultrafiltered volume may then be seen and precisely measured. With some modern automated machines, isolated UF may be difficult.

However, while technique has no limits, the human body has. The rapid removal of large quantities of fluid is a non-physiological interference and may cause serious problems. These will be described in Chapter 6, where the rather complicated dynamics of UF will also be discussed in detail. But even if these problems can be overcome it is very important to realize that a hemodialysis patient is never in a steady state. In some cases it will not be possible to remove the required amount completely and the patient will leave the dialysis session somewhat overhydrated. But this need not be the case. A frequent misunderstanding is that interdialytic weight gain is a measure of base-line overhydration. A patient can very well be continuously volume expanded, yet gain only little weight between dialysis sessions. However, if 'dry weight' is reached each time, his *average* weight during the week will be too high. There are two ways to avoid these large fluctuations: *salt restriction* and *more frequent dialysis.* These aspects are illustrated in Figure 2.3. From these considerations it is logical to diminish the need for UF by means of salt restriction, which prevents the accumulation of fluid. It can easily be calculated that if a patient gains 3 kg during two days and plasma sodium concentration remains normal, he has consumed 3 × 140 mmol or 13 g of salt per day, no matter how honestly he believes he is having a 'salt-free' diet.

It should be remarked that in a diabetic patient, changes in the body weight may not reflect salt balance. If blood glucose levels increase, thirst is stimulated and water is retained without salt. This will be reflected in a decrease in plasma sodium concentration.

Dietary salt restriction

For several reasons this highly desirable goal is often not reached.

The main difficulty of a low-salt diet is its *unpalatability.* The habit of salt consumption historically originates from the ability of NaCl to preserve foods. Later it became a cultural habit, which can best be characterized as a mild form of addiction. As with all addictions, people who are not used to it do not have that need, but once started find it difficult to abandon. The physiological background is that the taste threshold for salt adapts with time to the level of intake. People used to salted food may find a test solution tasteless, while people consuming a salt-free diet judge the same solution to be very salty. It takes several weeks at least for the taste sensation to adapt to a new level. If a patient, trying to keep to a salt-free diet, occasionally takes some salted food, the adaptation will not occur. Contrary

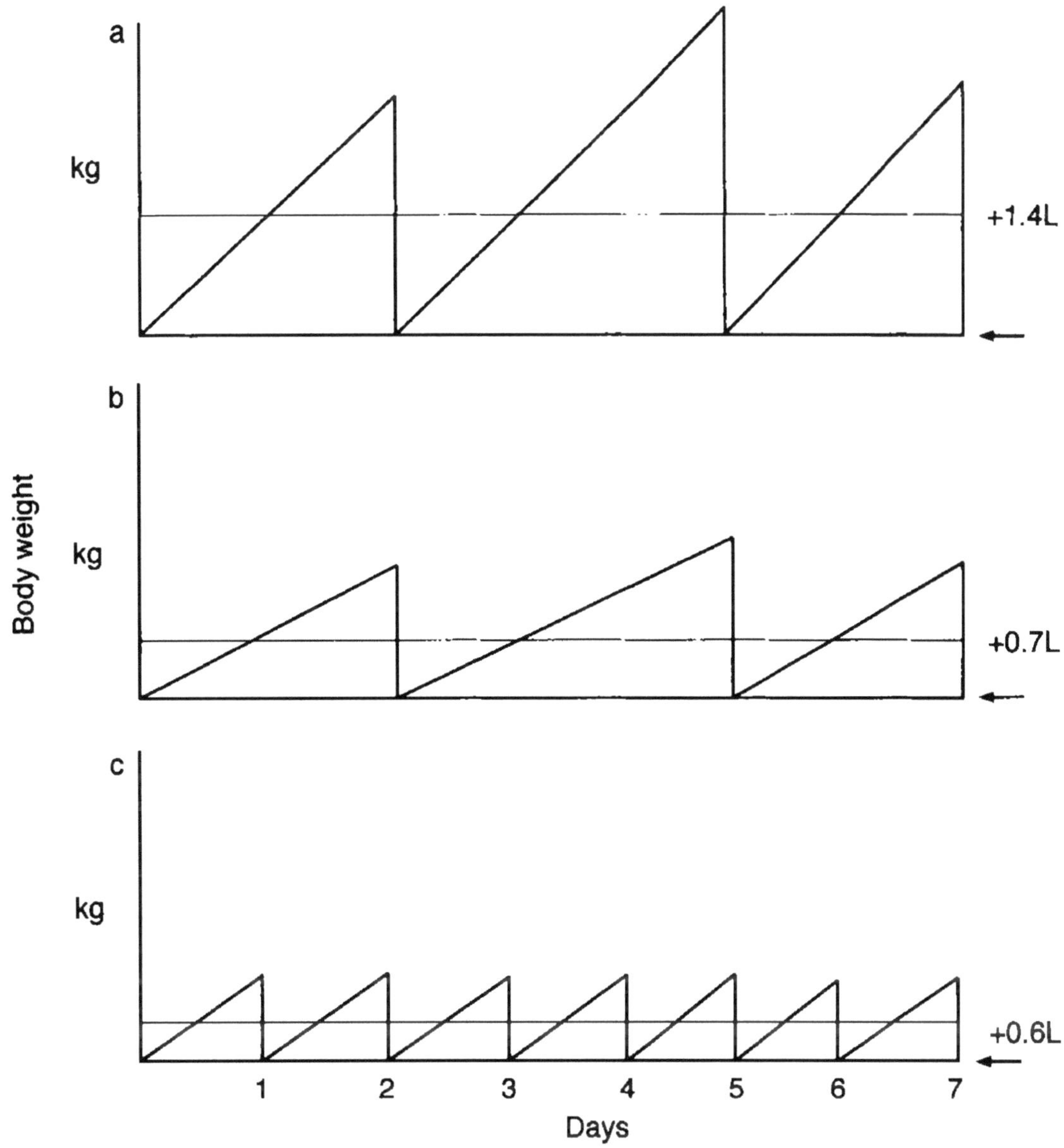

Figure 2.3 'Harmonica effect' Schematic presentation of weight (and thus volume) changes during a week hemodialysis treatment. (a) Usual situation: large gains due to salt consumption. (b) Smaller variations during salt restriction (5–6 g/day). (c) Unrestricted salt but daily dialysis. Note that, even if the bottom line represents the ideal ('dry') weight, the *mean* body weight during the week will be well above this value, indicating 1.4, 0.7 or 0.6 L fluid excess respectively.

to popular belief, spices like pepper, garlic, etc. are in no way harmful and their use can be encouraged in order to make the food tastier. However, some commercial herb mixtures contain large amounts of NaCl. Of course no 'salt substitutes' are allowed for dialysis patients as they contain other salts (K, Mg or NH_4) that may even be more harmful than NaCl. These facts have to be carefully explained in order to convince the patient. Just one 'pep talk' is not enough and the doctor or nurse should also try to speak and explain these things to the family member who prepares the food. An uninformed patient will be non-compliant. Non-compliance is a modifiable risk factor.

Studies on urea kinetics have shown that some dialysis patients have been undernourished. The introduction of membranes with better permeability and more frequent dialysis have made a more liberal protein diet both desirable and possible, but the continuing need for salt restriction is often not stressed. Rather the idea, 'Never mind, we will ultrafiltrate it off' has prevailed.

The main source of NaCl nowadays is prepared food. Efforts to make producers indicate the sodium content of their products have been unsuccessful, due to the political influence of the food and salt industries. In particular, bread contains a varying, unquantified amount of salt.

Thus a 'no added salt' diet is not sufficient to ensure the necessary sodium restriction.

Eating during dialysis

It is often suggested that the patient may eat a normal unrestricted meal during a dialysis session, because 'everything eaten will be washed out'. This is a serious misconception because it is well known that the time necessary for digestion and resorption exceeds the dialysis time. In contrast, after food consumption, digestive juices are drawn from the blood and secreted into the intestinal system. It has indeed been shown that eating increases the danger of hypotension during dialysis (Figure 2.4). In addition it has unwanted psychological effects, because it is difficult to convince a patient to keep to a diet, but make an exception three times a week.

Water restriction

Unfortunately, incomplete understanding of the principles of salt and water dynamics, explained in Chapter 1, may lead to the patient being advised to restrict water consumption, and reproached for too much drinking when there is excessive weight gain. The patient is also inclined to believe that gaining 3 kg means 3 L of water. While this is true, the *cause* of it is too much salt. Forcing him to drink less will not only fail to correct the volume overload, but also cause unbearable thirst. Thus the patient will not comply. Instead his attention will be drawn away from the real culprit, which is salt. It is sufficient to drink not more than his thirst feeling indicates. If a patient drinks too much water, hyponatremia will occur. This is not seen frequently, but if it happens it is important to know that it generally does not mean lack of salt, but abundance of water! In clinical practice hyponatremia is

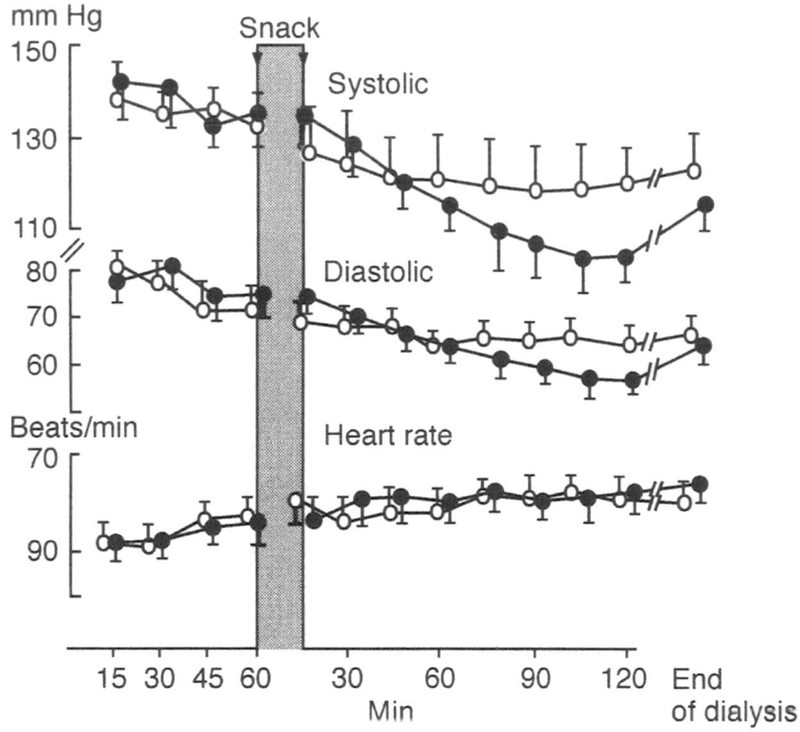

Figure 2.4 Arterial pressure and heart rate during control (○) and snack (●) hemodialysis. From Zoccali C et al. 1989, with permission.

mostly seen together with overhydration, and attempts to correct it by giving salt will only aggravate ECV expansion.

Having reviewed the main physiological principles and shown that fluid retention is a constant threat, we will discuss the pathophysiological consequences of volume expansion in the following chapters.

Summary

- Replacement of renal function by dialysis not only implies removal of waste products, but above all means keeping body fluid volumes normal.
- Efforts to improve the disappointing mortality figures have unfortunately been concentrated on urea removal (*KT/V* concept), neglecting volume control.
- Volume control is achieved by removing the accumulated fluid by ultrafiltration during the dialysis sessions. As a result, the hemodialysis patient is never in a steady state.
- Rapid fluid removal causes serious complaints and often does not reach the required goal.
- While longer and or more frequent dialysis sessions will improve the results, the most logical and effective measure is serious dietary salt restriction.

- Insistence on water restriction is ineffective, unnecessary and often counterproductive.
- Explaining the basic principles of salt and water to the patient is essential, because an uninformed patient is likely to be non-compliant.
- Non-compliance is a modifiable risk factor.

Bibliography

Charra B, Calemard E, Ruffet M et al. Survival as an index of adequacy of dialysis. Kidney Int. 1992;41:1286–91.

EDTA-ERA Committee: Report on management of renal failure in Europe XXIII 1992. Nephrol Dial Transplant. 1994;9(Suppl. 1):5.

Gotch FA, Sargent JA. A mechanistic analysis of the National Cooperative Dialysis Study (NCDS). Kidney Int. 1985;28:526–34.

Levey AS, Eknoyan G. Cardiovascular disease in chronic renal disease. Nephrol Dial Transplant. 1999;14:828–33.

Lowrie EG, Laird NM, Parker TF, Sargent JA. Effect of the hemodialysis prescription on patient morbidity. N Engl Med. 1981;305:1176–81.

Shaldon S, Koch KM. Are standards and checklists needed in uremia therapy? Kidney Int. 1985;28(Suppl. 17):124–26.

Schulman G. A consensus report on the dose of dialysis: Quantity and time. Am J Kidney Dis. 1998;32(Suppl. 4):86–87.

United States Renal Data System: 1989–1993. Annual Data Reports: The National Institute of Health, National Institute of Diabetes and Digestive and Kidney Diseases, Bethesda, MD.

Wizemann V, Kramer W. Short-term dialysis, long-term complications: ten years experience with short-duration renal replacement therapy. Blood Purif. 1987; 5:193–201.

Zoccali C, Mallamocy F, Ciccarelli M et al. Postprandial alterations in arterial pressure control during hymodialysis in uremic patients. Clin Nephr. 1989;31:323–26.

3

Results of fluid retention

Any increase in ECV that results from salt retention will lead to a cascade of events which are schematically summarized in Figure 3.1. We will analyze these developments step by step.

ECV EXPANSION LEADS TO BLOOD VOLUME EXPANSION

Terminology

Because blood volume (BV) and extracellular volume (ECV) are closely related, the terms fluid retention, overfilling and hypervolemia are not sharply defined and are often used interchangeably. We will use 'fluid retention' and overhydration for an increase in ECV and 'hypervolemia' for an increase in BV, while avoiding the word 'overfilling'.

Relation between ECV and BV

As the blood plasma is a part of the extracellular volume, plasma volume and therefore blood-volume (BV) change concomitantly with the ECV. For every liter ECV excess, BV would increase 180 ml (Figure 3.2). Because the

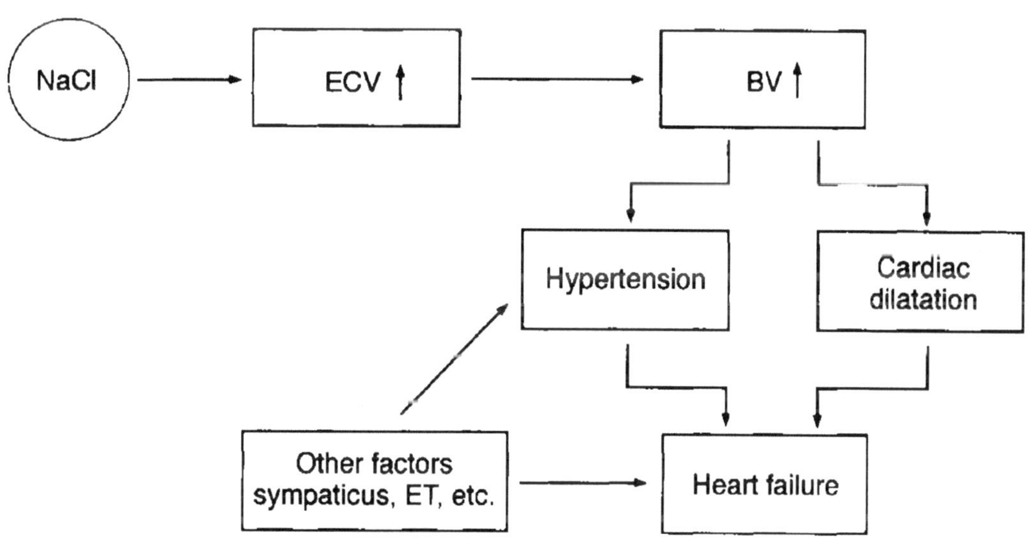

Figure 3.1 Short- and long-term consequences of salt retention.

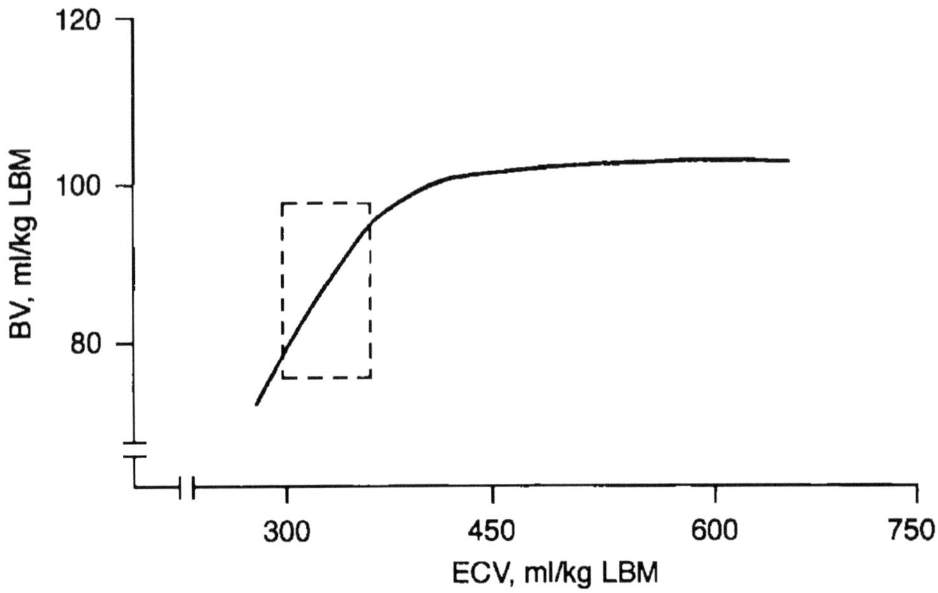

Figure 3.2 Relationship between extracellular volume and blood volume in patients with chronic renal failure. Adapted from Koomans et al. 1986.

'Starling forces' which govern the partition between BV and interstitial volume may change, this relationship is not the same in all circumstances. For instance, in patients with low plasma colloid osmotic pressure (like the nephrotic syndrome) BV hardly increases despite the large increase in interstitial volume.

A very important fact about the ECV–BV relationship is that it is *not linear.* This is also illustrated in Figure 3.2, which shows BV and ECV measured in patients with renal failure at different levels of fluid retention. BV increases only slowly when ECV expansion exceeds 5 L, which is the amount where edema appears. It is evident that the volume of blood within the vascular system cannot increase indefinitely, while there is no apparent limit to expansion of the ECV.

Compliance

The best way of describing the factors determining the distribution of volume excess is the *compliance* of the compartments. This is the ease or willingness to accept an increase in volume, a kind of elasticity. A high compliance indicates a high elasticity, while a low compliance means stiffness. Mathematically it is defined as the change in hydrostatic pressure (P) which occurs at a given change in volume (V): $\Delta P/\Delta V$.

Compliance may change in pathological conditions. For instance the interstitial space normally has a rather low compliance, because its pressure (which is negative) increases when the volume increases. This is due to the fact that interstitial fluid is not freely movable, but is in a gel-like form.

When edema appears, the gel structure is broken, compliance becomes very high and therefore many liters of fluid excess can accumulate without a measurable change in interstitial pressure. It is clear that the equilibrium between BV and IV depends on the difference between interstitial and intracapillary pressures. The precapillary vascular resistance and venous pressure determine the latter. The fact that the compliance of the interstitial and probably also of the blood compartment changes with expansion explains why the curve describing their relationship is not linear.

These considerations have important practical consequences. Because the curve is steepest close to the normal value, relatively small changes in ECV will affect BV most in that region. For example, ultrafiltration of 2 L in a patient with 5 L excess of ECV (which may not cause visible edema) will be easily tolerated, but if we reduce the volume of a patient with only 2 L excess to normal the BV of that patient will decrease twice as much as in the one with 5 L excess. Not much research has been done in this field. Consequently the effect of hematocrit, compliance of the different compartments of the vascular system and, above all, the functional condition of the heart have not been documented. These factors, which vary from patient to patient, should have an important influence on the BV/ECV relationship.

Acute changes

When we remove a large amount of excess fluid in a short time with ultrafiltration (UF) there will be a temporal *dysequilibrium* because time is needed before a new steady state is reached. Figure 3.3 illustrates that BV decreases excessively during UF after which a shift (refill) will take place. Not surprisingly, this temporary decrease in volume is also accompanied by a temporary decrease in blood pressure. This 'plasma refill' is larger when BV has dropped more, but also depends on the amount of ECV expansion. When there is a large fluid excess, the interstitium will easily permit a shift (large compliance). Of course, refill starts during UF but continues thereafter (see also Figure 6.3). While this process mainly takes place within one hour, the final adjustment may take 24 hours to be completed. These rather complicated adjustments are nicely illustrated by the graphic presentation of the treatment of the patient (Figure 3.4) who was admitted with severe overhydration: ECV excess + 11 L, BV excess + 0.8 L. During daily ultrafiltration the ECV was reduced stepwise to normal, but the BV shows a rebound after every session due to 'post-dialysis refill'. Note that the broken line indicates the relation between ECV and BV in the steady state (similar to Figure 3.2) while the increasing steepness of the lines during dialysis shows the decreasing refill rate when volumes approach normal values. These problems will be discussed in more detail in Chapter 6.

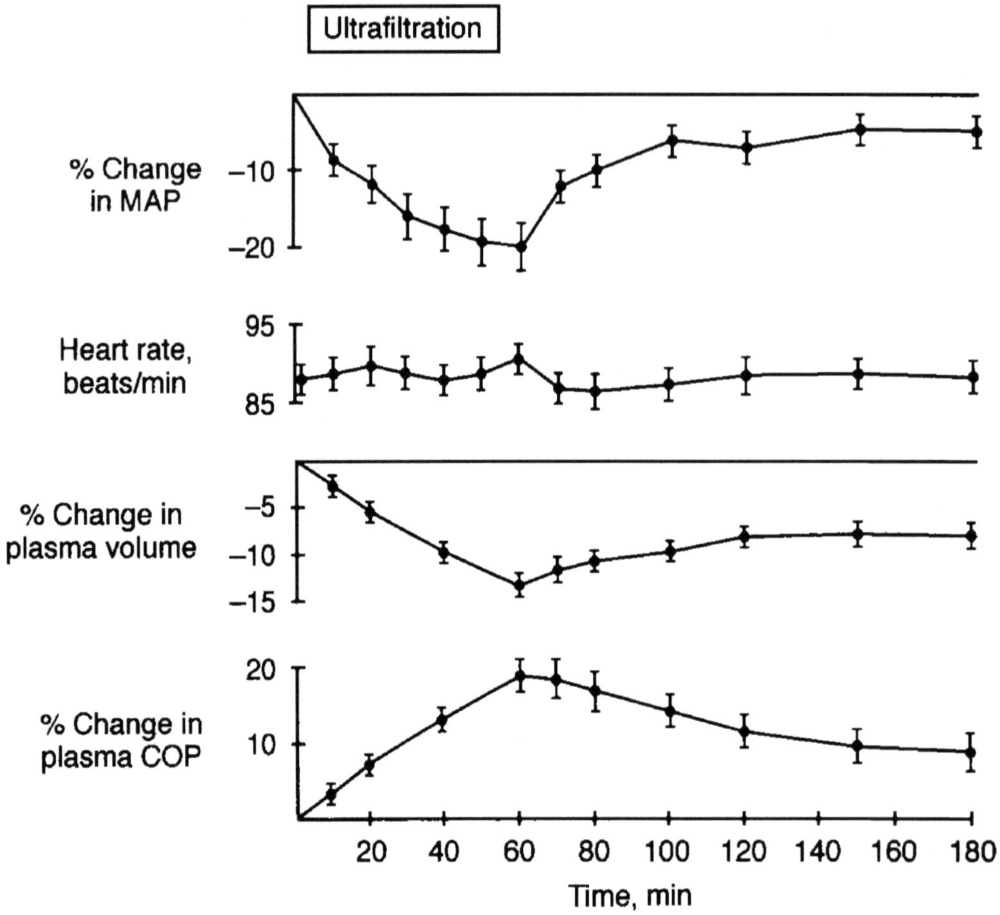

Figure 3.3 Changes in mean arterial pressure, heart rate, plasma volume and colloid osmotic pressure (COP) after 2 L ultrafiltration From Koomans et al. 1984 (Ch. 6), with permission.

2 CONSEQUENCES OF BLOOD VOLUME EXPANSION

Cardiac dilatation

The increased volume will be distributed within the cardiovascular system according to the relative compliance of its different compartments. In addition to their elastic properties these compartments also have muscular walls which may actively change their compliance. As the venous system has the largest compliance, this will expand first, with a small but important increase in pressure. This can be estimated echographically by an increase in diameter of the inferior vena cava (see below). At the same time more blood will reach the heart, leading to some increase of diastolic dimensions. This increase in cardiac volume can be easily proven by the fact that the diameter of the heart on the chest X-ray decreases 0.5–1 cm after a 'normal' 2–4 L fluid subtraction during dialysis. According to the Frank Starling law of the heart this hypervolemia must also lead to increased cardiac output

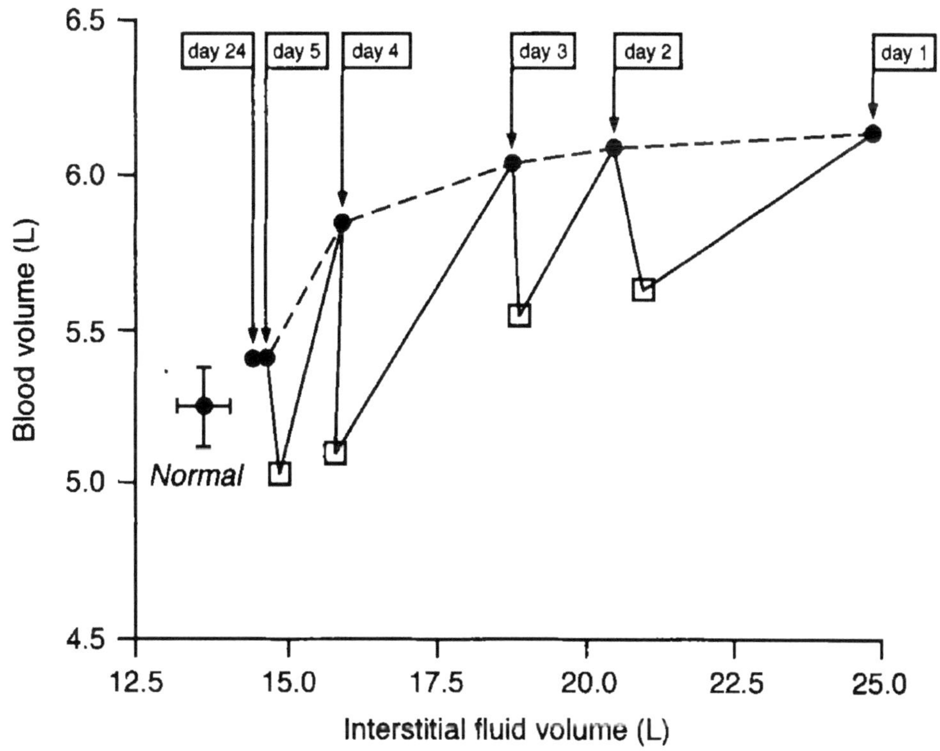

Figure 3.4 Changes in blood volume and interstitial fluid volume in an individual patient, who entered the hospital in overfilled state and was ultrafiltered daily. ● Prior to ultrafiltration, □ Immediately after ultrafiltration. See text for comments. Adapted from Koomans 1996.

and a *hypercirculatory state*. Because the normal volume regulation is absent, any volume retention beyond normal variations represents a constant burden. Depending on its magnitude it will lead to a variety of changes in shape, structure and function of the heart, which will be detailed in Chapter 8.

Hypertension

It is an undisputed fact that fluid retention, most probably by hypervolemia, leads to *hypertension* in many patients. An example is given in Figure 3.5, where the blood pressures of the same patient group shown in Figure 3.2 are plotted against the changes in ECV. The curve is also not linear and strongly resembles the BV–ECV relationship. The most plausible explanation as advocated by Guyton is that the hypercirculation causes hyperperfusion of the tissues. Thus the blood delivers more oxygen than their metabolism needs, which eventually leads to down-regulation of the blood flow by vasoconstriction. This *autoregulation* of the body tissues results in increased total peripheral resistance and hypertension (Hall et al. 1996). This sequence of events has not been proven in all patients, and not only

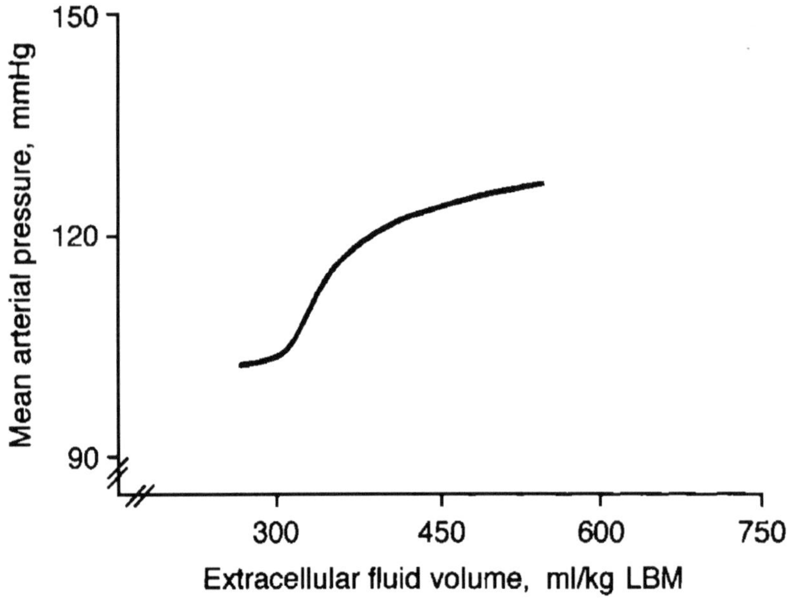

Figure 3.5 Relationship between extracellular volume and blood pressure, as measured in patients with renal failure at various degrees of fluid retention. Shape of the curve is similar to the one in Figure 3.2, suggesting that the determinant of blood pressure is the blood volume. Adapted from Koomans et al. 1986 (Ch. 6).

the autoregulation theory but also the relative importance of hypervolemia for dialysis hypertension is still being debated. Nevertheless the notion that overhydration is undesirable is not contested. It therefore is of crucial importance to know how much fluid excess is present in each patient.

3 THE 'DRY WEIGHT' CONCEPT

Definition

Dry weight is defined as the weight of a person whose *extracellular volume* is normal. With few exceptions a normal blood volume accompanies this, and consequently no signs should be present of either hypervolemia or hypovolemia as found upon physical examination or additional tests (see below). Dialysis is aimed at restoring this euvolemic condition by ultrafiltration, and the weight at which euvolemia is present is used as a guide during dialysis sessions. As will be explained in Chapter 6, the often used definition that 'dry weight is the weight below which hypotension occurs' cannot be a reliable guideline.

Changes in body weight between dialysis sessions reflect changes in ECV only when the (effective) osmolality does not change. As a decrease in plasma Na concentration indicates an excess of water in the intracellular compartment, the use of body weight as a guide will, in that case, cause an overestimation of the ECV.[1] In clinical practice Na concentration seldom shows important variations. In diabetic patients, however, a rise in glucose concentration will attract water and decrease plasma Na concentration. Indeed it was recently reported that only half of the interdialytic weight gain in diabetic patients was accounted for by sodium retention, the other half being due to hyperglycemia.

Because the unphysiological ultrafiltration method is used, achievement and maintenance of dry weight cause many problems. The fluid state of the patients is a rhythmic process (Figure 2.1) and focussing on a single end-point like post-dialysis weight basically cannot assess fluid dynamics adequately. With this reservation, the following methods can be used to estimate whether the patient is hypervolemic, euvolemic or hypovolemic. They include estimations of ECV as well as BV.

History and physical examination

Problems are particularly important when they occur in the interdialytic period and should be specifically enquired about. If fainting, hypotension and lassitude appear, the patient is probably hypovolemic and his target dry weight has been too low. In contrast, exertional and nocturnal dyspnea suggest increased pulmonary arterial pressure by overhydration and erroneously established too-high dry weight. Physical examination should include estimation of central venous pressure and looking for pitting edema, but many liters of excess fluid may be present without this classical sign. Despite their inaccuracy these methods should not be neglected because they are simple and, used routinely, may detect changes in condition of the patients which would otherwise be unrecognized.

Recently the usefulness of regularly applying a scored index of signs and symptoms was emphasized. Apart from correlating well with other methods it also revealed a surprisingly high number of dysvolemic periods necessitating adjustment in target dry weight (Wizemann and Schilling 1995).

Ancillary methods

The diameter and collaps index of the inferior vena cava just under the diaphragm measured by echography is a more sensitive method to estimate venous congestion. The diameter should be judged in relation to the body build and sex of the patient. With respiration, the pressure and thus the diameter in the vena cava change. The fractional decrease in diameter on inspiration is called the 'collaps index'. With hypervolemia pressure remains

---

[1] During dialysis, Na will diffuse to the blood and the amount to be ultrafiltrated will yet have to match the increase in body weight.

high and the collapse index remains close to 1. With hypovolemia it may completely collapse during inspiration. Normal value is 0.6. Both diameter and collapse index correlate with right atrial pressure. However, the method is fraught with technical problems and needs an experienced echographist and the collaboration of the patient. The site of measurement is critical and sometimes a good image cannot be obtained. Moreover the collapse index is influenced by the heart rate. Despite theoretical advantages, its value in predicting the fluid state of the individual patient is rather poor (Mandelbaum et al. 1993).

The volume of the heart can be most easily estimated by a chest X-ray. Although it has many inaccuracies it is still a useful, easy, but much neglected method. Efforts should be taken to let the patient stand up and inspirate adequately to enhance the accuracy of the X-ray. A cardiothoracic index of 0.48 or higher is pathological and most often indicates hypervolemia. More insight is of course given by *echocardiography* (see Chapter 7 for details).

Another valuable method is the blood level of *atrial natriuretic peptide* (ANP) (or its marker cyclic GMP) which reflects the pressure in the atria. It is a sensitive index of acute volume changes and useful for comparison. For instance it was found to be greatly elevated in a group of patients with 'untreatable' hypertension, showing that they were not – as was assumed on clinical grounds – on their 'dry weight' (Fishbane et al. 1996 (Ch. 5)). ANP may not decrease to completely normal levels despite achievement of normal intra-atrial pressure. While this has been interpreted as inappropriate, it may also be the result of stretching by chronic fluid overload. In that case, central venous pressure would not be an accurate reflection of the true volume status in some patients, and prolonged efforts to reduce volume further might be indicated. This important issue remains to be investigated.

ECV can be estimated by *bio-impedance.* This elegant method needs special apparatus and experience and has not been used routinely so far. Increased fluid content of the lung has been found with new techniques in HD patients.

The disadvantage of all these methods is that they need apparatus and time, and cannot be applied easily at the bedside. Moreover the moment of measurement in relation to dialysis is important. As remarked by Wizemann (1995), these indices when recorded during and post dialysis (as is often the case) 'might reflect rather an acute dysequilibrium between vascular and extravascular volume than euvolemia of the extra cellular space'. The tests should ideally be repeated regularly because the condition of many patients varies. In one study the target weight had to be adjusted three times a year per patient.

Finally short-term changes of ECV can be estimated from changes in body weight. Acute changes in BV during UF can accurately be measured by changes in Ht or plasma proteins. Recently, devices have become available to monitor these changes on-line during dialysis. The applications of these methods and the problems involved will be further discussed in Chapter 6.

Hypertension is a sure sign of overhydration in many patients, although the proportion of patients whose hypertension is due to factors other than hypervolemia vary considerably among investigators. Personal experience supported by data from the literature suggests that these discrepancies are mainly due to difficulties in achieving 'dry weight' over longer periods. Once convinced of the importance of overhydration a dialysis team will try harder and will be more successful. When it is assumed that hypervolemia is absent in a hypertensive patient he is usually treated with hypotensive drugs. Because these drugs interfere with the homeostatic regulation of blood pressure, they may aggravate blood pressure fluctuations during ultrafiltration. It has indeed been reported that the correlation between interdialytic weight gain and blood pressure is lost in patients using these drugs (Figure 5.3b) and that when a patient is on anti-hypertensive medication, achievement of dry weight is virtually impossible.

The major difficulty during attempts to achieve dry weight is attacks of *symptomatic hypotension* and muscle cramps during ultrafiltration dialysis. Contrary to general belief such attacks are no proof that dry weight has been reached.

There are three ways to facilitate achievement of dry weight: 1. *Longer dialysis sessions* enabling removal of fluid excess more slowly, or including a period of 'isolated' ultrafiltration without dialysis; 2. *More frequent sessions* to reduce the amount of fluid removed per session, and still reach the required total amount; 3. *More severe sodium restriction*. The common goal is to reduce the speed of blood volume reduction. By applying one or more of these methods, several groups have been able to achieve normotension without drugs in a large proportion of their patients. The notion that persistent or recurrent hypertension is one of the main indications that dry weight has not been reached is not shared by all investigators, however. The question whether or not unrecognized volume retention is responsible for most cases of hypertension in dialysis patients is probably the most important issue in dialysis treatment, because it has far-reaching practical consequences. In the early days of dialysis treatment, a much larger proportion of the patients were reported to be 'volume sensitive'. Some authors have suggested that the 'case mix' has changed, implying that other pathophysiological mechanisms are prevalent nowadays.

The volume–pressure relationships will be described in more detail in Chapter 5. Getting ahead of this discussion, it is helpful to mention that it often takes much *time* for the blood pressure to adapt to a new volume level. This 'lag phenomenon' implies that the BP will remain somewhat elevated when dry weight is reached and will come down gradually. This is illustrated in Figure 3.6.

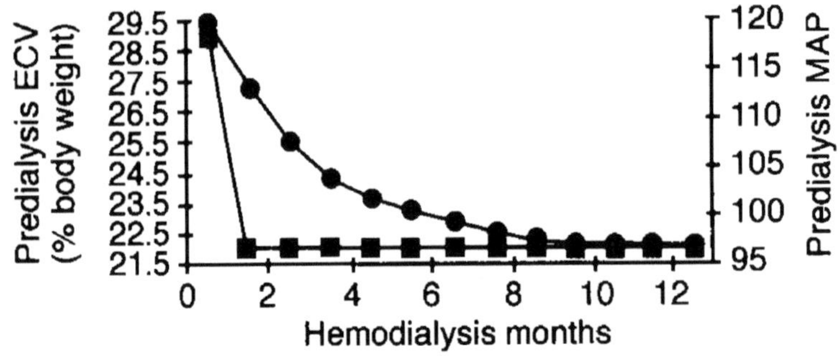

Figure 3.6 Theoretical graph of predialytic ECV (lower curve) and mean arterial pressure (MAP) (upper line) during the first 12 months of hemodialysis. From Charra et al. 1998, with permission.

A normal BP figure on the other hand, does not prove that there is no hypervolemia. Particularly in patients with long-standing cardiac damage and dilatation, blood pressure may be normal or low. In such patients volume reduction is difficult, but still possible and sometimes very beneficial (Chapter 8.5).

Summary

- ECV expansion leads to BV expansion, but the relation is not linear and depends on the changing compliance of both compartments.
- During acute changes by ultrafiltration (UF) BV 'lags behind' because 'plasma refill' takes time.
- BV expansion causes both blood pressure rise (hypertension) and cardiac dilatation.
- 'Dry weight' is the weight of a patient when all body fluid volumes are normal and is used as a guide for the desired amount of UF.
- Determination of dry weight is not easy, and basically is done by methods which estimate normovolemia. Episodes of collapse and muscle cramps during UF are no proof of normovolemia.
- Blood pressure is an important yardstick for normovolemia, and use of antihypertensive drugs makes achievement of dry weight very difficult.
- The opinion advanced in this book, that volume retention is responsible for more than 90% of hypertension in dialysis patients, is not shared by all investigators.

Bibliography

Charra B, Bergström J, Scribner BH. Blood pressure control in dialysis patients: Importance of the lag phenomenon. Am J Kidney Dis. 1998;32:720–24.

Hall JE, Guyton AC, Brands MW. Pressure–volume regulation in hypertension. Kidney Int. 1996;49(Suppl. 55):35–41.

Jaeger JO, Mehta RL. Assessment of dry weight in hemodialysis. J Am Soc Nephrol. 1999;10:392–403.

Koomans HA, Braam B, Geers AB. The importance of plasma protein for blood volume end blood pressure homeostasis. Kidney Int 1986; 30: 730–735

Koomans HA. Body fluid dynamics during dialysis In: Zoccali (ed). Clinical hypertension in Nephrology. Contr Nephrol. 1996;119:173–81.

Mandelbaum A, Link G, Wambach G, Ritz E. Vena cava ultrasonography assessing the state of hydration of patients with renal failure. Dtsch Med Wschr. 1993;118:1309–15 (English summary).

Schneditz D, Roob J, Oswald M et al. Nature and rate of vascular refilling during hemodialysis and ultrafiltration. Kidney Int. 1992;42:1425–33.

Tan SY, Nolan J, Craig K et al. Changes in atrial natriuretic peptide and plasma renin activity following changes in right atrial pressure in patients with chronic renal failure. Am J Nephrol. 1995;15:18–23.

Wizemann V, Schilling M. Dilemma of assessing volume state – the use and limitations of a clinical score. Nephrol Dial Transplant. 1995;10:2114–17.

4

Hypertension in dialysis patients

1 PREVALENCE OF HYPERTENSION

While hypertension occurs in ±15% of a normal population, its frequency is much higher in patients with renal disease. Roughly speaking the incidence increases in parallel with progression of renal failure, and by the time dialysis treatment is started, up to 90% of the patients are hypertensive. The appearance of hypertension is related to the nature of the renal disease. It is most frequent – and may start before functional impairment – in various glomerular diseases and polycystic kidneys, while its onset is later in primary tubular and interstitial disorders. This difference is probably due to differences in salt excretion impairment and/or in activity of the renin–agiotensin system. Once the patient has become anuric, the relation of BP to the underlying disease is less clear, but this subject has not been sufficiently analyzed.

When dialysis treatment is started and excess of body fluids is removed by UF, hypertension disappears in many patients during the first months.The first patient surviving on chronic hemodialysis (1960) suffered from malignant, seemingly intractable hypertension, but became normotensive (and remained so for 11 years) after aggressive ultrafiltration. Since then several studies have documented that around 90% of hypertension responds to strict volume control.

During the past years however, the incidence of hypertension among dialysis patients around the world has markedly increased and for that reason the dominant role of hypervolemia in its pathogenesis is being contested. In fact, although systematic registration is lacking, the available reports show large regional differences in prevalence. In one Italian center, hypertension decreased gradually from 80% to 40% of the patients during the first half year of treatment. The EDTA made a limited questionnaire in 1992: Pre-dialysis systolic BP was >140 in 70% of the patients and diastolic pressure >90 mm/Hg in 30%. The median BP was 145/85. In 1994 Health Care Financing Administration reported a mean BP of 152/79 mmHg in the USA (Figure 4.1). Based on an in-depth review of the literature the HCFA committee could not find 'enough data to submit an evidence-based clinical practice guideline'! Another study (Cheigh et al. 1993) from that country found blood pressures >160/90 in 62% of the patients and concluded 'that hypertension is not adequately controlled'. These figures are even more striking if one considers that the majority of the patients were treated with antihypertensive drugs. In sharp contrast, several other reports have shown

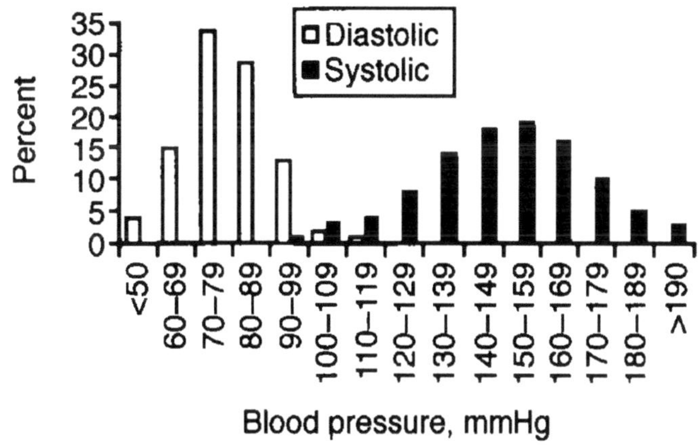

Figure 4.1 Distribution of predialysis systolic and diastolic BP values for adult hemodialysis patients in the USA. 1996 core indicator study. (From Mailloux et al. 1998, with permission).

much better BP values. These were from centers where much attention was given to volume control and salt restriction. In one (Uruguay) 72% of the patients had normal BP without drugs (MAP 89 ± 12 mmHg) the others had a mean MAP of 97 ± 9 (Fernandez et al. 1992). All of the patients (58% of the total) who were treated with long dialysis sessions in a center in the UK had normal BP (116/67) without drugs (Goldsmith et al. 1997). A Turkish center reported a mean BP of 131/80 ± 17/9 in all 67 patients treated with strict volume control during one year (Özkahya et al. 1999 (Ch. 5)). The most impressive results were obtained in Tassin (France) where BP could be normalized in 97% of the 712 patients (Carra et al. 1992).

The failure to achieve BP control by the great majority of dialysis centers around the world has led to speculation that the present-day type of patients ('case mix') is different from the past and also varies between populations. However, the extreme differences in BP control shown above make it much more likely that they are related to the *method of treatment*.

2 WHICH BLOOD PRESSURE IS REPRESENTATIVE?

When reading reports on BP in dialysis patients one gets the impression that the BP of such a patient can be easily determined, but everybody who regularly looks at patients' charts knows that this is not the case. Because of the intermittent nature of hemodialysis (and UF) the patient is never in a steady state. BP usually decreases during a session and gradually rises thereafter until the next one. But both the 'pre-dialysis' and the 'post-dialysis' values also vary from one session to the other. According to some reports, pre-dialysis BP may overestimate, while immediate post-dialysis BP may certainly underestimate the prevailing level.

In addition, the *day-to-night rhythm* of BP is lost in most patients with renal failure. Thus the 15–20% decrease in BP during the night that occurs in normal persons is absent. This means that these 'non-dipper' patients are exposed to higher levels of mean BP during 24 hours and are likely to suffer from more end-organ damage than estimated from their daytime values. Consequently, 24-hour ambulatory BP recording has been advocated to better determine the 'real' BP. The reason for the loss of circadian rhythm is obscure. It is not corrected by antihypertensive drugs, but may be partly related to overhydration. The proportion of non-dippers was less in the very strictly volume-controlled patients. This notion is supported by a recent report showing that sodium restriction restores circadian rhythm in non-dippers with essential hypertension (Fujü et al. 1999).

Keeping all these considerations in mind, it is probably not necessary to apply continuous recording in order to estimate a patient's risk. For clinical practice the mean of repeated inter-dialysis or pre-dialysis determinations can be used as a guide.

3 HOW BAD IS HYPERTENSION FOR HD PATIENTS

Previously, when no effective treatment of hypertension was available, the conviction prevailed that high blood pressure was an inescapable fate and that lowering it might even be harmful. German doctors found a nice expression for this comforting view: *'Erfordernishochdruck'* (necessary hypertension). Since then, the devastating effects of hypertension in non-renal patients have been amply documented. What is more, large trials have shown such decreases in morbidity and mortality after antihypertensive treatment that this may be considered one of the most important successes of modern medicine.

In *dialysis patients* hypertension was likewise considered to be a major risk factor for their high cardiovascular morbidity and mortality. Earlier reports mentioned increased CV complications with systolic as well as diastolic BP elevations. Later studies, however, with huge numbers of patients have concluded that hypertension has little or no relation at all to mortality! In one large study from the USA only systolic BP > 180 mmHg was associated with decreased survival. It was found that low blood pressure has a particularly bad prognosis (so-called J or U curve). Consequently it is being suggested that higher pressures be the aim in dialysis patients. A recent survey of 649 HD patients found an inverse relationship with survival over the entire BP range: patients with MAP ± 115 had 56% longer survival that those with MAP + 101! Strangely enough only black patients were better off with high blood pressure in that study (Salem 1999). Another author concluded that the association between predialysis hypertension and mortality was surprisingly small (Port et al. 1999).

In sharp contrast, a group of investigators (Charra et al. 1994), who applied meticulous volume control with long dialysis sessions, not only achieved better survival with good BP control than almost all other centers, but also found a significant reduction in death rates with lower BP values even within the normal range (Figure 4.2).

These diverging results seem rather confusing. Yet despite the fact that most of these studies accounted for other risk factors and used sophisticated statistical analyses, it is clear that *confounding factors* must have caused these discrepancies. The most plausible explanation for the bad prognosis of patients with low-to-normal blood pressure is the *condition of the heart* (Figure 4.3). It is well known that heart failure is associated with decrease in blood pressure. It was shown recently that the 'J'or 'U' curve seen in elderly patients with essential hypertension can be explained by the fact that previously high BP decreases before the patient dies from heart failure. Unfortunately, none of the multi-center studies which may suggest that hypertension is not harmful in dialysis patients provides information on the condition of the heart. However, the authors of one study (Foley et al. 1996) suggest that a similar explanation of this paradox applies to dialysis patients: BP fell when heart failure developed, and heart failure pre-dated most deaths in their study.

Indeed, hypertension is a major contributor to well-established risk factors such as increases in left ventricular mass index and volume as well as atherosclerosis, ischemic heart disease and de novo cardiac failure in dialysis patients. Therefore it is likely that hypertension itself is involved in the development of these complications. In patients with essential hypertension, the diluting effects of random fluctuations in BP have caused substantial underestimation of the association with stroke and coronary heart disease (MacMahon et al. 1990). Considering the fact that individual fluctuations

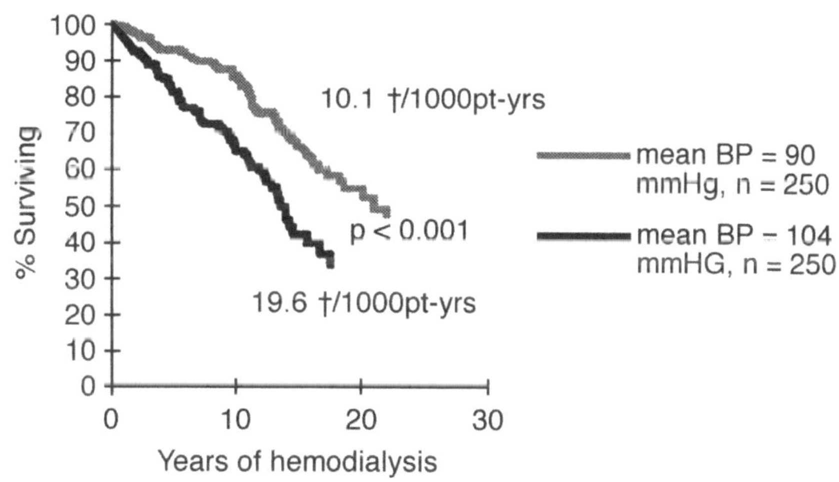

Figure 4.2 Survival and cardiovascular mortality in two patient subgroups up and down the median predialysis BP. (From Charra 1994, with permission).

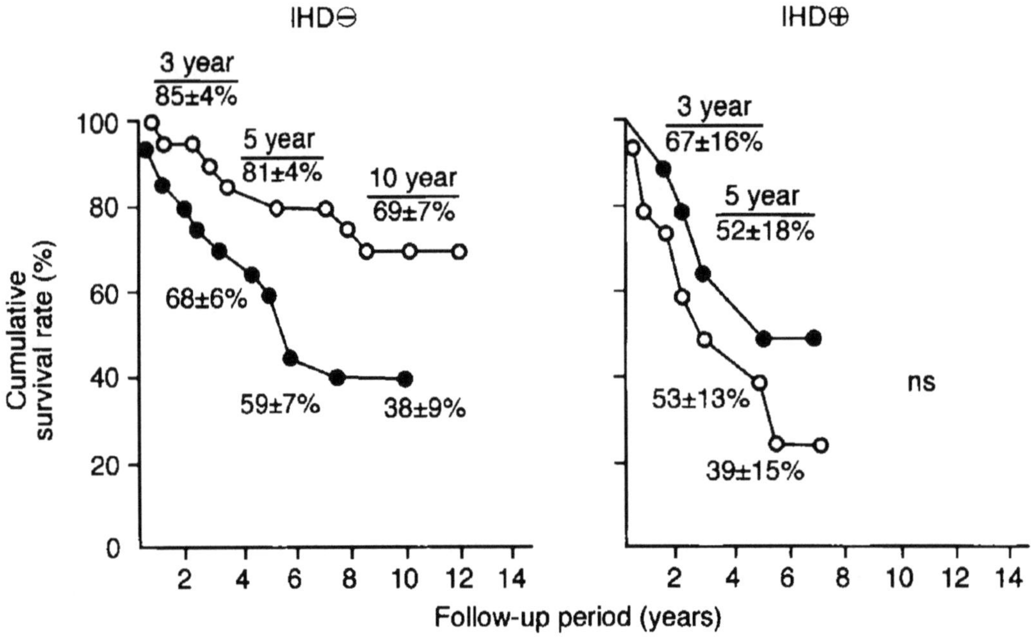

Figure 4.3 Different impact of blood pressure on survival in hemodialysis patients depending on the presence or absence of ischemic heart disease (IHD). ○ Systolic BP < 160 mm Hg. ● BP > 160 mm Hg. (From Kimura 1996, with permission).

are very much accentuated in dialysis patients, one would expect that such 'regression-dilution bias' is even more important in this group.

After all, hypertension is a long-term process, and observations during dialysis describe only a late phase. The assumption that a simple linear relationship between hypertension and mortality is also present in short-term studies neglects the complicated nature of these problems. Despite the fact that the available data leave a lot of questions, far-reaching consequences have followed the studies that did not substantiate the positive relationship between cardiovascular death and blood pressure. In contrast to the overwhelming body of research on the pathophysiology and treatment of hypertension in general, stands the scarce attention given to hypertension in the dialysis patient. Probably conflicting data on this subject have discouraged investigators.

The main aim of the present book is to intensify the focus of the reader for this highly interesting problem, which can be approached with pathophysiological rules of volume and pressure control. With the harmful effects of hypertension on cardiovascular morbidity in mind, the analysis in this book will provide clues to the treatment of this *preventable* abnormality, which requires the attention of the whole dialysis team.

4 WHAT IS THE OPTIMAL BLOOD PRESSURE?

Before engaging in treatment, an important question to be answered is the level of BP that should be aimed at. Some authors advocate to lower BP to

160/90 or below, others suggest upper limits of 150/90 and 140/80. The finding in some studies that low BP is associated with increased mortality in dialysis patients may discourage any serious attempt to lower BP. Assuming that the J curve is due to an artifact, renal patients will be considered as not basically different from patients with essential hypertension and diabetes. In those groups a continuous relationship between BP and cardiovascular complications is present with no clear lower limit. This would imply that *complete normalization* is the ultimate aim. This is supported by the findings of Charra et al. mentioned above.

This does not mean that BP should be lowered immediately to normal values in all patients. As will be explained in Chapter 5, it takes time for the body to adapt to a new BP level, particularly when the heart has been damaged. Good clinical judgment is indispensable and therefore close supervision of the patient during this adjustment period is necessary.

It should also be remarked that dialysis patients have, for several reasons, a high pulse pressure with elevated systolic pressure while diastolic pressure is often in the 'normal' range. At variance with traditional teaching, systolic elevation carries the most important risk in these patients. (see Chapter 9).

In conclusion, these considerations would imply that BP in dialysis patients should be lowered on a short-time basis below 145/85 and eventually to 125/80 or even lower during the following 12 months.

Summary

- Hypertension is almost invariably present in end-stage renal failure.
- Dialysis enables withdrawal of excess fluid by UF, which often results in normalization of BP.
- In recent years the incidence of hypertension among dialysis patients has increased and the pathogenic role of volume expansion is contested.
- However, in several centers around the world, good BP control is achieved, suggesting that the differences are related to the way of treatment.
- In sharp contrast to patients with essential hypertension, no correlation between the level of BP and mortality was reported in some studies on dialysis patients.
- Excess mortality in the low-BP group is probably due to pre-terminal BP drop caused by a bad condition of the heart.
- Arguments are presented to normalize BP despite some uncertainties.

Bibliography

Charra B. Control of blood pressure in long slow hemodialysis. Blood Purif. 1994;12:252–58.

Cheigh S, Milite C, Sullivan JF et al. Hypertension is not adequately controlled in hemodialysis patients. Am J Kidney Dis. 1993;19:453–5993.

Coomer RW, Schulman G, Breyer JA et al. Ambulatory blood pressure monitoring in dialysis patients. Am J Kidney Dis. 1997;429:678–84.

Fernandez JM, Carbonell ME, Marzuchi N et al. Simultaneous analysis of morbidity and mortality factors in chronic hemodialysis patients. Kidney Int. 1992;41: 1029–34.

Foley RN, Parfrey PS, Harnett JD et al. Impact of hypertension on cardio-myopathy, morbidity and mortality in end-stage renal disease. Kidney Int. 1996;49:1379–85.

Fujü T, Uzu T, Nishimura M et al. Circadian rhythm of natriuresis is disturbed in non-dipper type of essential hypertension. Am J Kidney Dis. 1999;33:29–35.

Goldsmith DJ, Corvic AC, Venning MC et al. Ambulatory blood pressure monitoring in renal dialysis and transplant patients. Am J Kidney Dis. 1997;29:593–600.

Kimura G, Tomita J, Nakamura S et al. Interaction between hypertension and other cardiovascular risk factors in survival of hemodialysis patients. Am J Hypertens. 1996;9:1006–12.

MacMahon D, Petro R, Cutler C et al. Blood pressure, stroke and coronary heart disease. Part 1, prolonged difference in blood pressure bias. Lancet. 1990; 335:765–74.

Mailloux LU, Haley WE. Hypertension in the ESRD patient. Am J Kidney Dis. 1998;32:705–19.

Port FK, Hulbert TE, Wolfe RA et al. Predialysis blood pressure and mortality risk in a national sample of maintenance hemodialysis patients. Am J Kidney Dis. 1999;33:507–17.

Salem MM. Hypertension in the hemodialysis population: any relationship to 2 year survival? Nephrol Dial Transplant. 1999;14:125–8.

Zager, Nikolic J, Brown RH et al. 'U' curve association of blood pressure and mortality in hemodialysis patients. Kidney Int. 1998;54:561–9.

5

Pathophysiology and treatment of hypertension in dialysis patients

In the preceding chapters the relationship between 'volume' and blood pressure has been mentioned several times. We will now discuss this and other factors involved in dialysis hypertension in more detail.

1 VOLUME EXPANSION

Autoregulation concept

Dialysis patients are constantly threatened by fluid overload and it would therefore be remarkable if most of them did not suffer from some hypervolemia. We saw in Chapter 1 that, according to Guyton, every increase in blood volume (BV) resulting from retention of extracellular fluid volume (ECV) should lead to elevated blood pressure (BP). The basic pathophysiological principle of this volume–hypertension concept is that the body tries to maintain fluid homeostasis at the expense of an elevated BP. Increased BV leads to a slight increase in right atrial pressure. A normal heart reacts to this increased 'pre-load' according to the Frank–Starling law by increasing cardiac output (CO). This *hypercirculation* induces vasoconstriction in the tissues (so called autoregulation), which increases BP further (Hall et al. 1996).

$$\text{ECV}\uparrow \Rightarrow \text{BV}\uparrow \Rightarrow \text{CO}\uparrow \Rightarrow \text{BP}\uparrow \Rightarrow \text{vasoconstriction} \Rightarrow \text{BP}\uparrow/\text{CO}\downarrow$$

Although a hypercirculatory state is present in many dialysis patients it is not easy to prove that this is caused by fluid overload because of confounding factors like *anemia* and A-V fistulas. It is even more problematic to prove that this also leads to hypertension along the sequence shown above. While one author described these events in a dialysis patient, others did not detect an increase in cardiac output when BP rose after overhydration, while in some patients BP did not increase at all (Kim et al. 1980). Nevertheless, whenever hypertension develops after volume expansion, it is always characterized by an increase in total peripheral resistance. This basic fact is often neglected in discussions on this subject, leading to the erroneous statement that the 'cause' of a patient's hypertension is in the arterioles. This, in turn, leads to a search for vasoconstrictive substances and the use of drugs that cause vasodilatation.

Subjects with normal kidneys do not show an increase in BP when they change from a salt-free to a salty diet. Only 50% of patients with hypertension experience an important change in BP when their salt intake is changed. Among the reasons for this difference, the reaction of the kidney is probably the most important one: The salt-excreting capacity of the kidney decides to what extent salt consumption results in volume increase. If it happens, only a small increase in volume (1–2 L ECV, within normal limits) can make the difference between normo- and hypertension. The renin–angiotensin system plays a modulating role. In patients with little or no renal function, however, every increase in salt intake invariably causes *volume expansion* and nearly always hypertension.

Features of BV–BP relationship

The volume–BP relationship has two very important features. The first is that it is not linear (see Chapter 3, Figure 5), implying that while a small increase triggers a BP rise, a larger volume excess may not cause a further rise. Thus, if a hypertensive dialysis patient has an ECV of 4 L above normal (which may not cause visible edema), the decrease of his weight by 3 kg with UF may not normalize his BP, leading to the wrong conclusion that he is 'volume insensitive'. As will be discussed in Chapter 6, removing the last liter of volume excess is much more difficult than removing the first liter.

Quite a different situation may arise when the heart is dilated and functionally impaired by long-standing hypervolemia. This may lead to a decrease in blood pressure. Decreasing the dilatation by ultrafiltration will then improve cardiac function and increase BP. This sometimes presents itself as paradoxical hypertension (see below). Another mechanism disturbing the volume–BP relationship may be *diastolic ventricular interaction* in which the dilated right ventricle hampers left ventricular filling.

The second feature of the BV–BP relationship is that *time* is needed before BP adapts to a change in BV. This time varies considerably from one patient to the other and it may take weeks or months before the new BP level is reached. Patients may remain slightly hypertensive after normovolemia has been achieved with UF, but show a gradual further decrease in BP when this volume is maintained. During this period body weight may actually increase due to an anabolic state which is illustrated in Figure 5.1. A laborious process of 'probing for dry weight' is necessary during the first weeks of treatment in new patients. This requires continuous efforts by the dialysis team (see also Figure 3.6). Similar results have been reported with *daily hemodialysis* by at least three groups of investigators. Also, with *conventional* dialysis times combined with severe salt restriction and occa-

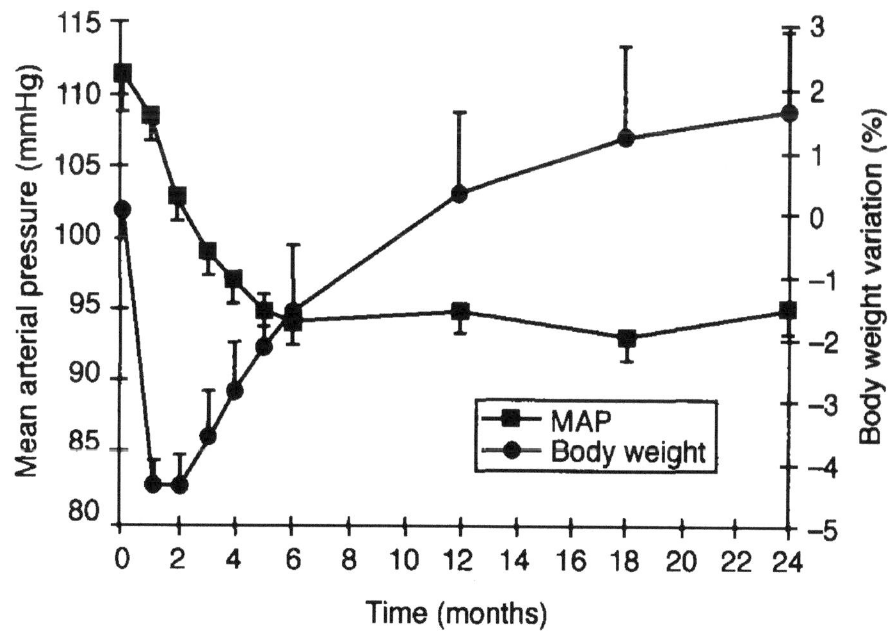

Figure 5.1 Changes in body weight and mean arterial pressure with time in a group of patients. Note the rapid drop in body weight due to removal of overhydration at the start of treatment, followed by a gradual rise due to increased dry weight by anabolism. In contrast, blood pressure further decreased during the first six months (from Chazot et al. 1999, with permission).

sional additional UF sessions, normotension could be reached in 67 hypertensive patients with only three of them using drugs (Özkahya et al. 1999). In the beginning hypotensive episodes are frequent, but they disappear once blood pressure has stabilized. The length of the time interval needed to reach complete normovolemia is probably related to adaptations of the dilated cardiac compartments. In these patients, CTi decreased from a mean of 0.54 to 0.47 after 12 months while MAP decreased from 120 to 103 mm Hg despite antihypertensive drugs being stopped in most cases (Figure 5.2).

A similar 'time lag' has been reported after diuretic treatment in hypertensive patients with normal kidneys but it seems that the lag period is longer in (some) dialysis patients. This slower adaptation may be related to less flexible regulating mechanisms, but probably also to 'remodeling' of the dilated, hypertrophied heart and blood vessels. It is clear that this lag phenomenon very much complicates achievement of normal blood pressure.

It also seems that it takes less time for hypertension to develop than to regress. Although the few days between two dialysis sessions are too short to reach a steady state, 90% of the patients have a rise in BP during this time, the more so if their BP is already elevated. A factor confounding the relationship is the use of hypotensive drugs (Figure 5.3). In view of these facts it is not surprising that there are large differences between the reported frequencies of hypertension in dialysis patients and consequently between

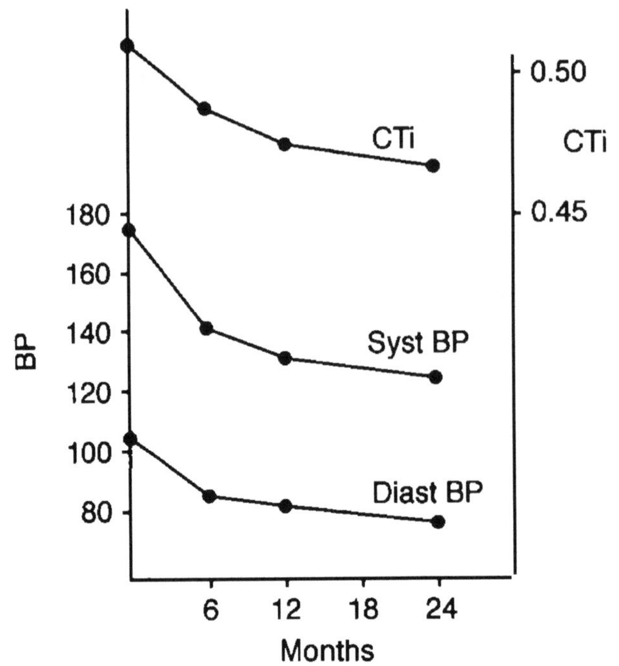

Figure 5.2 Gradual decrease in blood pressure during long term volume control, parallel with decrease in cardiothoracic indexes (CTi) (Data from Özkahya 1999.)

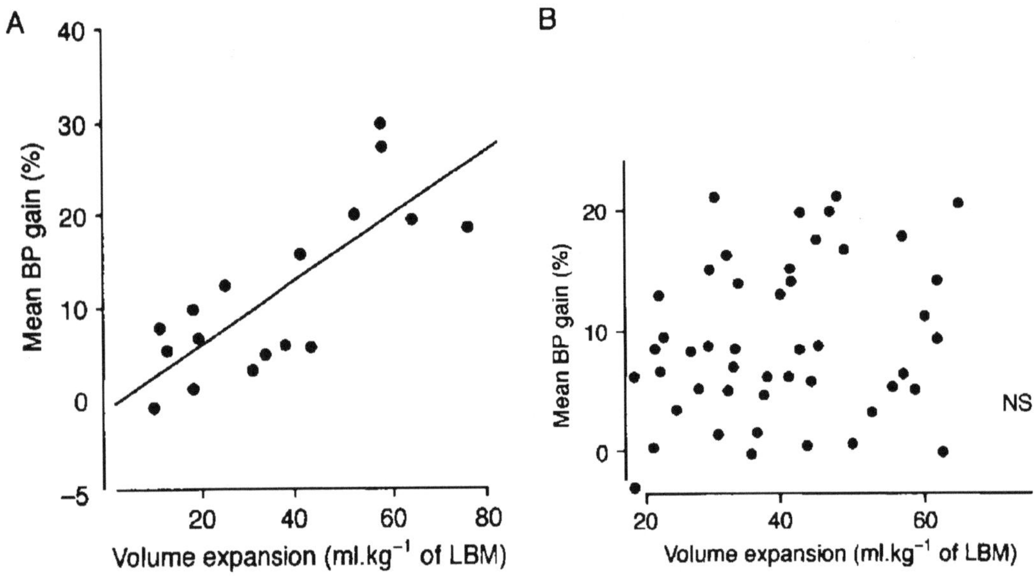

Figure 5.3 A: Relation between interdialytic volume gain and increase in blood pressure (BP). B: No such relationship in drug-treated patients (from Ventura et al. 1997, with permission).

the estimates by the authors on the pathogenic role of volume retention. The curvilinear relationship and the time factor can easily explain apparent contradictions in the literature, in particular the absence of a clear relationship between BP and short-time weight changes reported by some, but not by others. On the other hand, when groups of dialysis patients in a steady state were compared, those with hypertension usually had higher values for vena cava diameter, extracellular fluid volume, ANP levels or cardiothoracic index than those with normal BP, showing a clear relationship between volume status and BP (Katzarski 1997).

In conclusion, there is convincing evidence that hypervolemia is an important reason for the fact that a large proportion of dialysis patients still remain hypertensive. An argument for this contention is also the extreme variability of hypertension incidence among different dialysis centers. The autoregulation concept may act as a model in understanding the hypertension. Although this is still controversial, alternative explanations have not yet been proposed. The characteristics of the volume–blood pressure relationship (increased *peripheral resistance, non-linearity* and *the time factor*) make it understandable that this relationship often goes unrecognized. Nevertheless, *other factors* are operative and may play a contributory role.

2 RENIN ANGIOTENSIN SYSTEM (RAS)

The RAS is undoubtedly very important in the regulation of BP in normal man and in some hypertensive patients. In HD patients, renin secretion by the non-functioning kidney is not completely abolished and sometimes may be inappropriately high. In such cases, hypertension is resistant to volume control but may be lowered by bilateral nephrectomy or renin-lowering drugs, in particular angiotensin antagonists or converting enzyme inhibitors (CEI). Unfortunately, hardly any systematic, long-term investigation has been performed on this subject and as a result contradicting conclusions have been drawn which are difficult to reconcile with each other.

Because renin acts as a hormone and is subject to feed-back regulation in normal man, it is plausible to assume that this regulation must be disturbed when normal function and structure of the regulating organ are completely lost. Indeed available reports indicate that changes in plasma renin activity (PRA) which occur in normal persons upon changes in posture and volume are absent or diminished in dialysis patients. In particular, PRA is not influenced by the dialysis procedure. However, not unexpectedly there seem to be differences in sensitivity of the renin secretion to UF between individual patients (Figure 5.4).

How much does the RAS contribute to the maintenance of (elevated) BP in dialysis patients? Several reports have indicated that PRA is too high in relation to the volume status of hypertensive patients and that their BP can be related to the product of (log) PRA and volume. However, others could not confirm this contention. While some authors consider that the contribution of the RAS to BP is minor, others conclude that it plays an important role in nearly every dialysis patient. The latter view is strengthened by the fact that bilateral nephrectomy decreases BP in most patients including

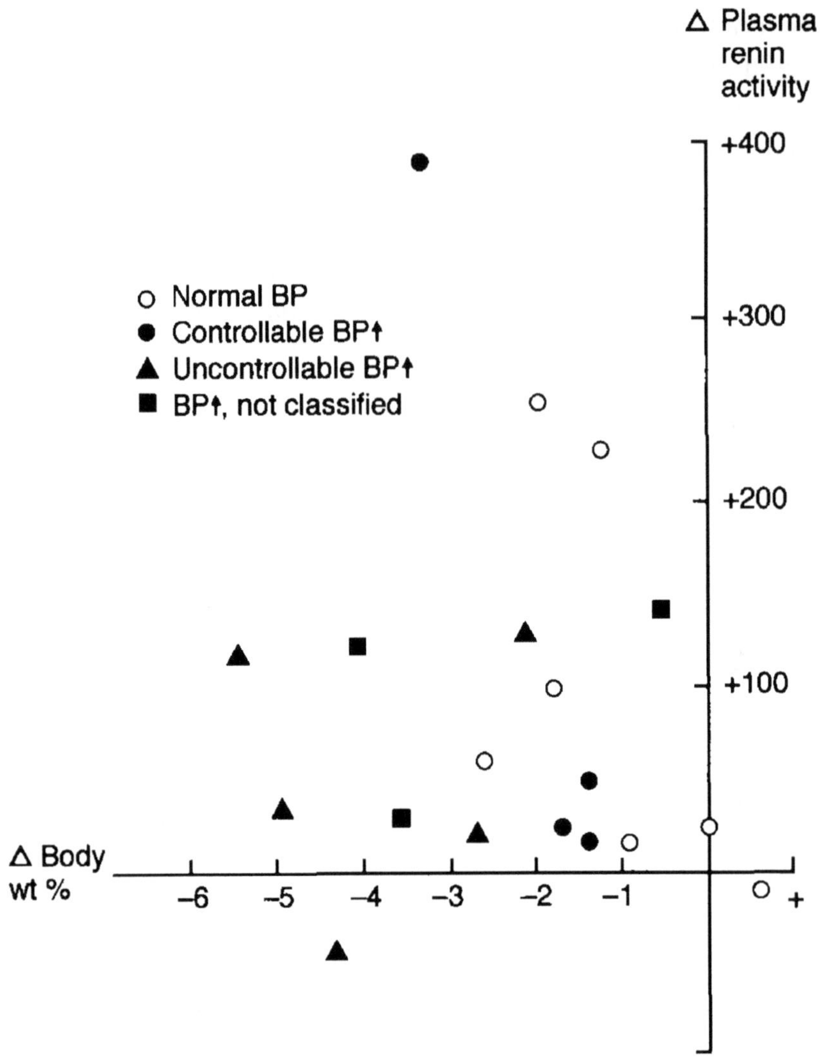

Figure 5.4 Absence of relationship between changes in body weight and plasma renin activity following hemodialysis (from Weidmann 1975, with permission).

those whose PRA is not elevated. The observation that in transplanted patients, persistent renin secretion by the diseased kidney contributes to hypertension, is a similar argument. On the other hand the influence of the RAS seems to be minor so long as overhydration is present. We systematically studied the acute effects of captopril in hypertensive dialysis patients and never observed a significant drop in BP as long as some volume expansion persisted. In a series of patients with advanced renal failure and not on dialysis treatment, the majority responded well to captopril, but right atrial and pulmonary artery pressures were normal in these patients, indicating the absence of overhydration (Schon et al. 1988). In *essential hypertension* captopril lowers BP also in a large proportion of the patients. It thus appears that during dialysis treatment the RAS contributes less to the maintenance of BP. It sometimes happens that a previously normotensive patient becomes hypertensive again during dialysis treatment (Figure 5.5). This is almost certainly due to fluid overload, because spontaneous increase in renin secretion by non-functioning kidneys has never been described.

Part of the explanation for these divergent views is probably the large variability between individual patients. In some dialysis patients vascular reactivity to vasoconstrictive stimuli, including angiotensin, are diminished (see Chapter 4). In addition, as the basic feedback regulation is certainly disturbed, decrease in renin secretion by the non-functioning kidney

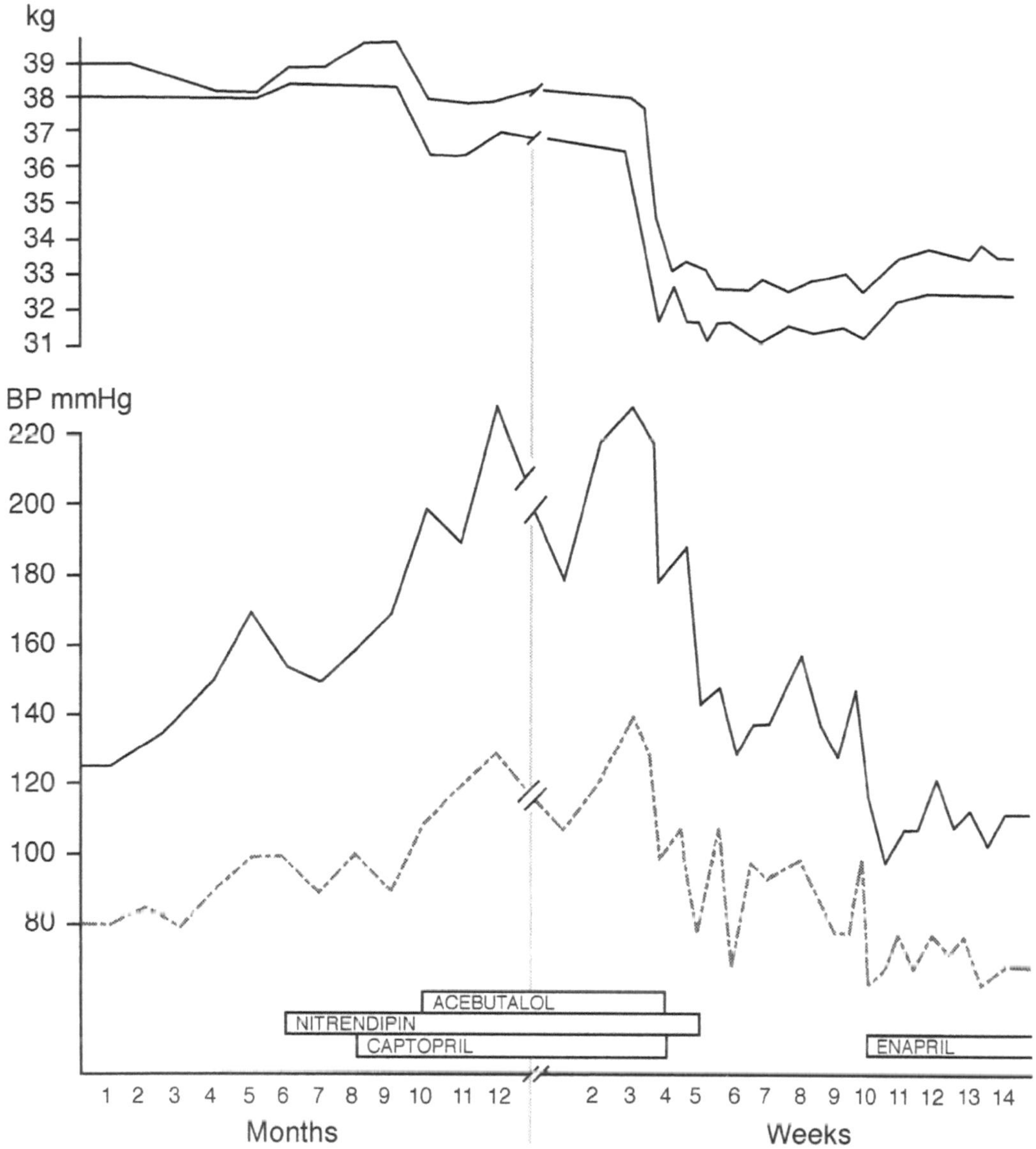

Figure 5.5 Development of malignant hypertension, resistant to multiple drug treatment that was corrected by ultrafiltration. When normovolemic, the patient became responsive to (previously ineffective) converting enzyme inhibition. Upper scale: body weight. Lower scale: systolic and diastolic blood pressure (from Ok et al. 1995, with permission).

appears an attractive hypothesis. This would partly explain the 'time lag' observed in the treatment of dialysis hypertension. Further research is urgently needed.

3 OTHER HYPERTENSIVE MECHANISMS

Besides 'volume' and 'renin', several abnormalities have been detected in dialysis patients and suggested to be responsible for their hypertension. In order to prove this assertion, it is necessary to provide evidence that the two well-known mechanisms, volume and renin, cannot explain the existing BP level. This is not easy and has never yet been done, but several interesting observations should be mentioned.

Sympathetic system

Just as in essential hypertension, much has been done in the past to find signs of increased sympathetic activity responsible for the increased BP in dialysis patients. Most tests, in particular measurement of plasma catechol-aminies, have yielded negative or equivocal results. However, the large decrease in BP observed after pharmacological sympathetic blockade provided indirect evidence for a role of this system. This was confirmed by the use of a new technique: direct measurement of sympathetic nerve discharge (SND). Converse et al. found that SND in HD patients was 2.5 times higher than in healthy control subjects. Remarkably, bilateral nephrectomy was associated with normalization of sympathetic tone. Thus sympathetic activation seemed to be mediated by an afferent signal arising in the diseased kidney. SND was unrelated to plasma norepinephrine levels, confirming that they constitute an inadequate tool to measure sympathetic activity. There was also no correlation between SND rate and PRA. On the other hand, Ligtenberg et al. showed that chronic (but not acute) CEI inhibition decreased SND together with BP in CRF patients not on dialysis treatment. Cardiac congestion is also accompanied by increased SND which decreases with treatment. Some of Converse's patients had severe hypertension and may well have been overhydrated. It thus cannot yet be concluded with certainty whether or how much increased SND contributes to hypertension.

Circulating substances

Elevated levels of blood-pressure-increasing factors have been detected in the blood of HD patients and implicated as causes of their elevated BP levels. Among these are endogenous digitalis-like substance, endothelin-1 and asymmetric dimethyl arginine (ADMA) The latter is an inhibitor of the synthesis of the potent local vasodilator *nitric oxide* (NO) and is insufficiently cleared by the dialysis procedure. Insufficient production of vasodilating factors like prostacycline has also been suggested as contributing to hypertension. As yet no proof has been provided for any of these hypotheses.

4 PARADOXICAL HYPERTENSION

When volume is reduced by ultrafiltration, the most frequent complication is an excessive decrease in blood pressure. In some patients however BP rises despite UF, even to frightening levels. For this unexpected increase the term 'paradoxical hypertension' is used. The first explanation which comes to mind is an 'overshoot' of the counter-regulating mechanisms, in particular the renin–angiotensin system, activated by the sudden decrease in volume. This explanation is usually accepted without much proof, but seems less likely because the reactivity of the renin system is diminished in dialysis patients. If renin were responsible for such crises it should be possible to prevent them by CEI treatment. Substantial evidence supporting this view is not available (Dorhout Mees 1996). In contrast, patients were described with paradoxical hypertension which was not prevented by CEI treatment. All of them had cardiomegaly, sometimes with functional valvular insufficiency. After more vigorous, repeated UF their BP decreased, intradialytic rises subsided and cardiac volumes and functions improved (Figure 5.6). Hypervolemia thus appears to be an important factor in this phenomenon. While explanations remain speculative at present, we hypothesize that the decrease in blood volume caused by ultrafiltration may improve cardiac output and functions when the heart is strongly dilated. Indeed as shown in Table 5.1, the decrease in volume during ultrafiltration was accompanied by a rise in the previously decreased ejection fraction. Thus hypervolemia may set the stage for paradoxical BP increases which subside when it is corrected. Unfortunately, the term 'hypovolemic hypertension' is sometimes used and this discourages the search for possible hypervolemia. Hypertension aggravated by volume depletion has been sporadically described in experimental malignant hypertensive rats and in one patient. Such rare cases respond to CEI and should not constitute a therapeutic problem. For clinical practice the most important message is that neglected fluid balance causes not only interdialytic hypertension but also 'paradoxical' rises during dialysis.

5 TREATMENT WITH ANTIHYPERTENSIVE DRUGS

As we saw in Chapter 4 the majority of dialysis patients both in the USA and in Europe are treated with antihypertensive drugs. However, long-term

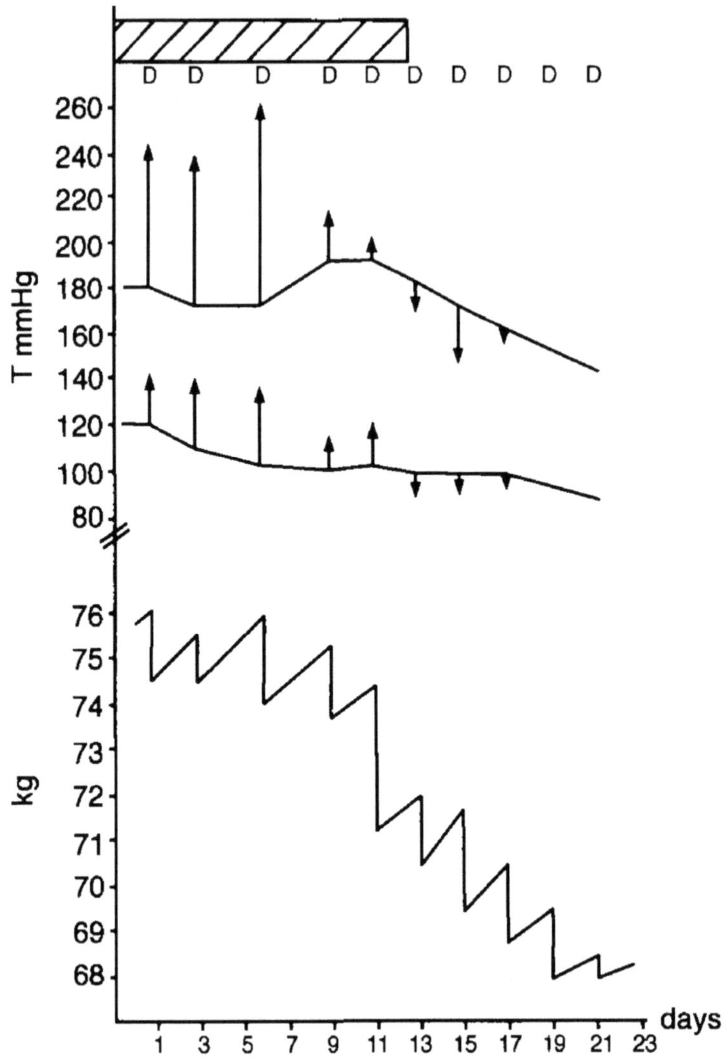

Figure 5.6 A patient showing 'paradoxical' rises in blood pressure (indicated with arrows) which disappeared after a weight loss of 7 kg. Hatched area indicates treatment with a converting enzyme inhibitor, D = dialysis-UF session. Lines represent systolic BP, diastolic BP and body weight. (from Cirit et al. 1995, with permission).

prospective trials are scarce and their ineffectiveness is seldom checked by temporary withdrawal of the drug. Such a control procedure is certainly needed because of the variability of BP in HD patients whose volume status is changing continuously. Likewise, controlled studies to identify the best drugs in hypertensive patients on dialysis are lacking. Textbooks list all drugs available on the market. Consequently there are very large variations in drug prescription. While in the very few centers applying rigorous volume control, fewer than 5% of the patients receive antihypertensive drugs, the mean consumption varied from 60% to 100% in European countries. In the USA the number of drug prescriptions has increased in recent years (Figure 5.7).

Table 5.1

	Body weight		Blood pressure		Left atrium diam. mm		Ejection fraction %	
Treatment	before	after	before	after	before	after	before	after
HD + UF	54	52	143/98	184/134	42	38	28	40
UF	53	51	160/80	190/100	45	38	24	47
HD + UF + C	55	52	180/100	200/100	44	36	24	47

Data of a patient with 'paradoxical hypertension' before and after three successive treatment sessions. HD = hemodialysis, UF = ultrafiltration, C = 50 mg captopril given immediately before session. Note that atrial diameter decreased and EF increased each time. After two weeks of intensified UF, his body weight decreased to 45 kg and cardiothoracic ratio from 0.62 to 0.46. His blood pressure stabilized at 130/80 mmHg and no paradoxical increases occurred any more.

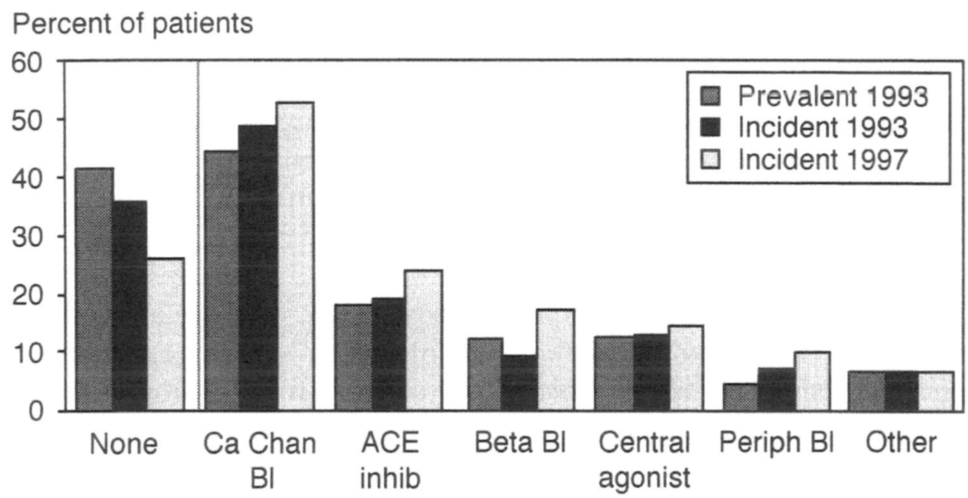

Figure 5.7 Increase in antihypertensive drug prescription in HD patients in the USA from 1993 to 1997. USRDS report 1998.

Calcium channel blockers are by far the most popular. Nevertheless, studies documenting their long-term effectiveness are few. One placebo-randomized study (London et al. 1990) showed that nitrendipine lowered blood pressure during a six-month period and was even more effective in patients with fluid retention. Its action was accompanied by a decrease in aortic pulse wave velocity and increased ejection fraction. This suggests a hypercirculatory state, which is indeed to be expected when vasodilatation is superimposed on hypervolemia. Thus while the pressure load on the heart is decreased, the volume load is increased. Indeed, no decrease in left ventricular hypertrophy was found (see also Chapter 8.2 on LVH).

Strong vasodilators are another option, and Minoxidil has been advocated in patients with refractory hypertension. However, in patients with essential hypertension it was shown to increase cardiac volume, muscle mass and ultimately morbidity (Leenen et al. 1990).

Converting enzyme inhibitors (CEIs) and angiotensin II antagonists are a logical choice for patients who are resistant to volume correction and probably have high plasma renin activity. Moreover CEIs also decrease sympathetic nerve discharge and have a favorable action on arterial and myocardial hypertrophy. However, if BP does not decrease after CEIs, they should not be continued, because this indicates that volume correction is necessary. CEIs may cause a severe anaphylactoid reaction when used in patients dialyzed with AN 69 membranes. This side-effect is not present with angiotensin blockers like losartran, but the anti-hypertensive effect of this drug is not better than that of converting enzyme inhibitors. A study using *losartran* reported only a mean decrease of pre-dialysis BP from 163/88 to 155/84 mmHg after three months.

In patients with heart failure and normal kidneys without hypertension, CEIs have been shown to be beneficial, but there is no proof that this also applies to dialysis patients. Although their direct action on the tissues of heart and arteries has been much stressed during the past years, this effect is marginal when compared to that of lowering blood pressure.

Beta-blockers may be the most effective choice (Agarwall 1999) according to the limited reports on drug treatment of hypertension in dialysis patients. Their mode of action comprises the decrease in renin secretion, the lowering of sympathetic activity and the reduction of cardiac output. In addition they have an anti-arrhythmic action.

The universal use of multiple drugs suggests that they are applied rather uncritically. Reports showing that patients using the highest number of drugs also have the highest blood pressures leave the impression that antihypertensive medication is often not effective (Sulkova and Valek 1988). The habit of using the number of antihypertensive drugs as an estimate of severity of hypertension is particularly deplorable. This is also illustrated in Figure 5.5.

In conclusion, the place of antihypertensive drugs is very limited in dialysis patients. If used inappropriately not only are they ineffective, but they also make volume control more difficult. By giving the treating team the comforting feeling that 'something is being done', attention may be diverted from the necessary volume control. But in dialysis patients, *drugs cannot correct volume.* In selected patients, beta-blockers or converting enzyme inhibitors are the most logical choice, but their blood-pressure-lowering effect must be clear, and recurrent overhydration prevented.

Summary

- Volume expansion is the most important cause of dialysis hypertension.
- The blood volume–hypertension relationship has the following characteristics: peripheral vascular resistance is increased, small volume increases

have the largest influence on BP, and time is needed for full expression of the relationship.

- The contribution of the renin–angiotensin system to hypertension in dialysis patients is not completely elucidated. A small number of patients whose BP is resistant to volume correction need angiotensin-lowering drugs.
- Other blood-pressure-increasing factors, notably increased sympathetic activity, are present in dialysis patients, but their role in blood pressure regulations is not yet clear.
- 'Paradoxical' hypertension during dialysis is often due to overhydration and cardiac dilatation.
- Antihypertensive drug treatment is mostly ineffective in dialysis patients because these drugs cannot correct volume overload.

Bibliography

Agarwall R. Supervised atenolol in the management of hemodialysis hypertension. Kidney Int. 1999;33:667–74.

Blumberg A, Hegstrom RM, Scribner BH. Extracellular volume in patients with chronic renal disease treated for hypertension by sodium restriction. Lancet. 1967;I:69.

Chazot C, Charra B, Vo Van C et al. The Janus-faced aspect of 'dry-weight'. Nephrol Dial Transplant. 1999;14:121–4.

Cirit M, Akcicek F, Terzioglu E et al. The cause of 'paradoxical' rise in blood pressure during ultrafiltration in dialysis patients. Nephrol Dial Translant. 1995;10: 1417–20.

Converse RL, Jacobsen TN, Toto RD et al. Sympathetic overactivity in patients with chronic renal failure. New Eng J Med. 1992;327:1912–18.

Dorhout Mees EJ. Rise in blood pressure during hemodialysis-ultrafiltration: a paradoxical phenomenon? Int J Artif Organs 1996;19:569–70.

Fishbane S, Natke F, Maesaka JK. Role of volume overload in dialysis-refractory hypertension. Am J Kidney Dis. 1996;28:257–61.

Hall JL, Guyton AC, Brands MW. Pressure–volume regulation in hypertension. Kidney Int. 1996;49(Suppl. 55):35–41.

Hinojosa-Laborde C, Frohlich BH, Cowley AW. Whole body auto regulation in reduced renal mass hypertension. Hypertension. 1992;20:659–65.

Katzarski S, Nisell J, Randmaa I et al. A critical evaluation of ultrasound measurement of inferior vena cava diameter in assessing dry weight in normotensive and hypertensive hemodialysis patients. Am J Kidney Dis. 1997;30:459-65.

Kim KB, Onesti G, DelGuercia ET et al. Sequential hemodynamic changes in end-stage renal disease and anephric state during volume expansion. Hypertension. 1980;2:102–19.

Leenen FHH, Tsoporis J. Cardiac volume load as a determinant of the response of cardiac mass to antihypertensive therapy. Europ Heart J. 1990; 11(Suppl. G): 100–6.

Ligtenberg G, Blankestijn PJ, Oey PL et al. Reduction of sympathetic hyperactivity by enalapril in patients with chronic renal faillure. N Engl J Med. 1999;340:1321–8.

London GM, Marchais SJ, Guerin AP et al. Salt and water retention and calcium blockade in uremia. Circulation. 1990;82:105–13.

Ok E, Akcicek F, Dorhout Mees EJ et al. Malignant hypertension in a haemodialysis patient treated by ultrafiltration. Nephrol Dial Transplant. 1995;10:2124–5.

Özkahya M, Toz H, Unsal A et al. Treatment of hypertension in dialysis patients by ultrafiltration: the role of cardiac dilatation and 'time factor'. Am J Kidney Dis. 1999;34:218–21.

Rahman M, Dixit A, Donley V et al. Factors associated with inadequate BP control in hypertensive dialysis patients. Am J Kidney Dis. 1999;33:498–506.

Schon DC, Jahn JH, Schmidt RL. Predictability of a standardized captopril test in hypertension in end-stage renal failure. Kidney Int. 1988;25:145–8.

Sorof JM, Brewer ED, Portman RJ. Ambulatory blood pressure monitoring and interdialytic weight gain in children. Am J Kidney Dis. 1999;33:667–74.

Sulkova S, Valek A. Role of antihypertensive drugs in the treatment of patients on regular dialysis. Kidney Int. 1988;34:198–200.

Ventura JE, Sposito M. Volume sensitivity of blood pressure in end-stage renal disease. Nephrol Dialysis Transpl. 1997;12:485–91.

Vertes V, Cangiana JL, Berman LB et al. Hypertension in end-stage renal disease. NEJM. 1969;280(18):978–81.

Weidmann P, Maxwell MH. The renin-angiotensin–aldosterone system in terminal renal failure. Kidney Int. 1975;8:S219–34.

6

Dialysis hypotension

1 GENERAL CONSIDERATIONS

Episodes of symptomatic circulatory collapse occur in 25% of dialysis sessions. They not only compromise the patients well-being, but also interfere with the attempts of the dialysis team to reach and maintain dry weight. Basically there is nothing mysterious about dialysis hypotension (DH). Depending on the state of overhydration, the removal of 2–4 L of extracellular fluid is accompanied by a 10–30% decrease in blood volume in a few hours. It can be imagined that circulatory adaptation to this unphysiological change may occasionally fall short of complete compensation. It is logical therefore, that the occurrence of DH will be greatly enhanced by two events: 1. *Insufficient dietary salt restriction causing excessive fluid gain* and 2. *Short dialysis.*

Salt intake

As shown in Chapter 2, a weight gain of 2–3 kg within 2–3 days (which is often considered acceptable) points to a sodium consumption of at least 140 mmol or 9 g salt per day, thus a 'normal' Western diet. And many patients gain more! But the more salt is eaten the more volume is retained. If a patient gains too much in the interdialytic period, episodes of DH will prevent ultrafiltration of this amount, and the average weight during the week will exceed his dry weight so much that hypertension and cardiac damage will be inevitable.

Factors which may have contributed to the world-wide negligence of salt restriction are unjustified emphasis on water instead of salt restriction and increased awareness of the need of a diet with adequate protein and calories without attention to salt. Unfortunately it takes quite some time to convince patients of the vital importance of salt restriction. The earlier this is done, the more effective it will be. While a dietician is of invaluable help, the doctor and nurse are primarily the persons who have to explain the reasons for it in simple terms and make them feel responsible for their own health, in order to prevent a 'naughty child' behavior.

Short dialysis

The availability of high-permeability membranes made it possible to remove urea and other waste products more quickly. Moreover, frequent short dialysis sessions are also more efficient in this respect. Thus pre-occupation with urea removal led to the habit of short dialysis sessions and short total dialysis time. While more frequent sessions will decrease the absolute amount of fluid to be removed during one session, the rate of fluid removal also influences DH. It appears that when the ultrafiltration rate exceeds 0.35 ml/kg/hour, acute blood pressure drops cannot be avoided.

2 SYMPTOMS OF DIALYSIS HYPOTENSION

Typically, DH occurs unexpectedly towards the end of the dialysis session. Two types can be distinguished: a *tachycardia* and a *bradycardia* collapse (Figure 6.1). The onset is always sudden in both types and due to an autonomic reflex (see page 60) The main symptoms are dizziness, drowsiness (up to black-outs), headache and muscle cramps. *Nausea* and *vomiting* are frequent in the *bradycardia* type. This distinction may not be that absolute and transitional forms exist. Older patients and diabetics are more prone to suffer from attacks of hypotension. These are not without danger and may precipitate cerebral and cardiac accidents.

Muscle cramps

Muscle cramps often accompany DH and are an innocent, but very unpleasant painful complication. They usually involve the lower leg muscles and occur regularly in about 25% of haemodialysis patients. Like similar cramps, which occasionally plague normal persons during the night, their pathophysiology is obscure. There is no doubt that this phenomenon is triggered by ultrafiltration and therefore usually arises during the second half of a dialysis session and during the hours after dialysis. Occurrence of muscle cramps is related to the speed of ultrafiltration and is no proof that all excess fluid had been removed.

Muscle cramps are neurogenic. Electromyography measurements have shown that they are preceded by a progressive rise in tonic activity, culminating in the paroxysm of the cramp. The mechanisms leading to this event are still being debated. Tissue hypoxia due to vasoconstriction or change of hemoglobin affinity for oxygen related with the transient alkalosis has been implicated, but cramps are not a usual feature of tissue hypoxia. Carnitine deficiency has been proposed as another not very likely candidate.

Acute relief of muscle cramps can often be obtained by intravenous fluid administration. Hypertonic solutions of glucose, mannitol or NaCl appear to be equally effective on an equimolar basis, but isotonic solutions may be as useful. Though hypertonic solutions allow a lower volume, they attract water so that unwanted ultimate volume expansion is not elleviated.

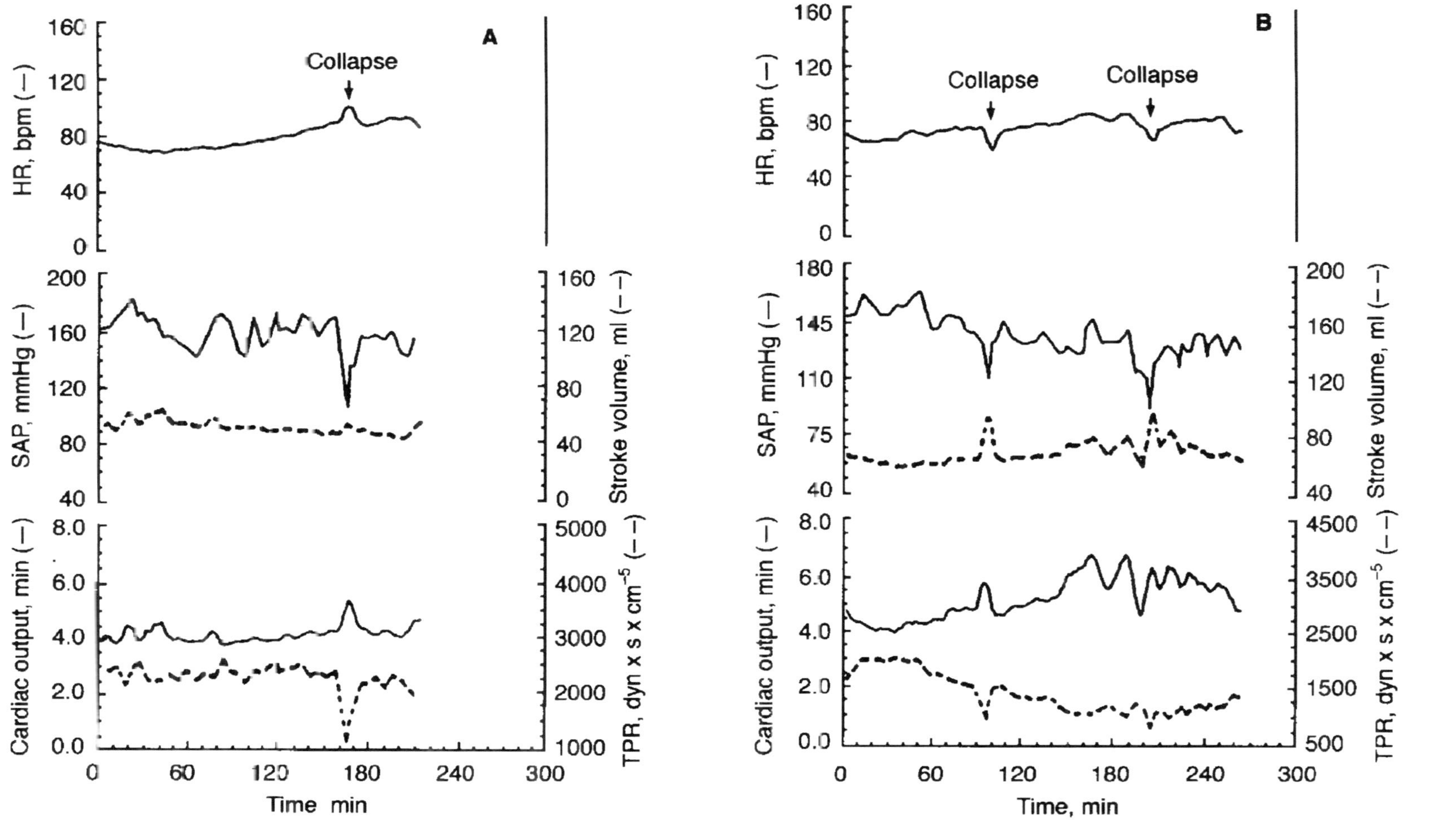

Figure 6.1 Circulatory changes during tachycardia (left) and bradycardia (right) attacks of dialysis hypotension. Note that both are accompanied by a sudden drop of total peripheral resistance (TPR) while cardiac output and stroke volume increase (from Santoro et al. 1990, with permission).

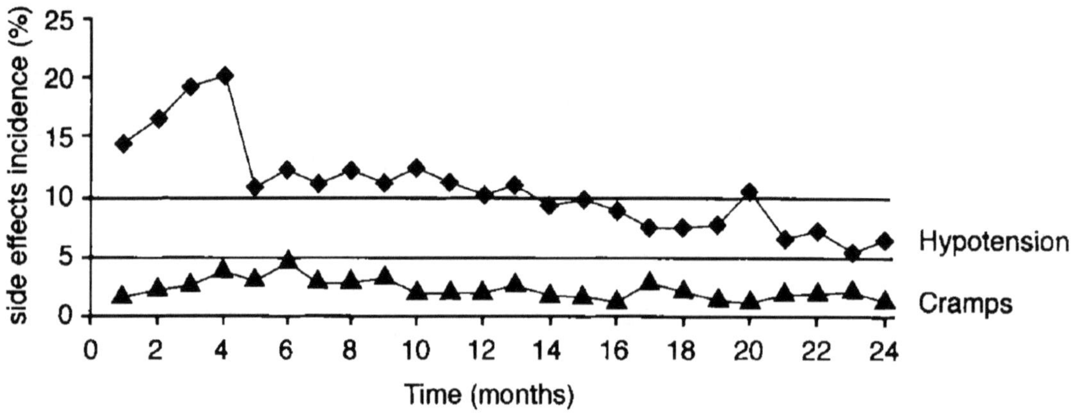

Figure 6.2 Gradual decrease in frequency of DH and cramps in a group of patients kept at their dry weight (from Chazot et al. 1999 (Ch. 4), with permission).

Preventive effects have been observed in oral quinine (325 mg). The effect of other suggested treatments, like carnitine, is not convincing. Vasodilating drugs such as prazosin and nifedipine have been proposed but do not seem suitable for a complaint which is particularly associated with hypotension. Finally it has been suggested that psychological factors are also influential. As shown in Figure 6.2, the incidence of hypotensive episodes and muscle cramps decreases with time if dry weight and normal blood pressure are maintained.

3 PATHOGENESIS OF DIALYSIS HYPOTENSION

The mechanism of DH is (nearly) always a decrease in circulating blood volume with a decreased filling pressure of the heart. This causes a reflex with acute withdrawal of sympathetic activity resulting in circulatory collapse (see page 60 for details on cardiac function). Theoretically, there are several possibilities why the latter could happen: (1) too much fluid may be removed, the patient became hypovolemic; (2) the ultrafiltration rate exceeds the physiological compensatory regulation; (3) the dialysis procedure interferes with normal circulatory adaptations; (4) the 'uremic state' impairs compensatory mechanisms.

Too much ultrafiltration

Too much fluid may have been removed because 'dry weight' has been erroneously determined to be too low. Some authors claim that excessive UF beyond dry weight is the main cause of DH. This can certainly happen, particularly in patients who are normotensive. We should be aware of this possibility because dry weight may increase unnoticed in well-dialyzed patients because of improved nutrition.

Dynamics of ultrafiltration: the crucial role of refill

During UF both the (increased) intravascular and the extravascular volumes decrease. Although the equilibrium between these two compartments is established fairly rapidly, this process still needs some time. As the ultrafiltrate is withdrawn from the blood, there will be a *fluid shift* from the interstitium to the plasma called 'plasma refill'. The main motive force is the *increase in oncotic pressure* of the blood caused by the removal of protein-free filtrate. It is clear that refill will be minimal at the start of UF and increase as 'inspissation' of the blood progresses, until refill rate equals UF rate (Figure 6.3). When UF is stopped, refill will continue for some time until complete equilibration of the new steady state. Thus, to achieve normovolemia after establishment of a new equilibrium between interstitium and plasma, a hypovolemic situation at the end of the dialysis session may be inevitable. In other words, if we want to make a patient's blood volume normal, we have to make him hypovolemic for a short time!

The 'Starling forces' at the capillary level determine the refill process. The increase in oncotic gradient will decrease the net fluid flow from the

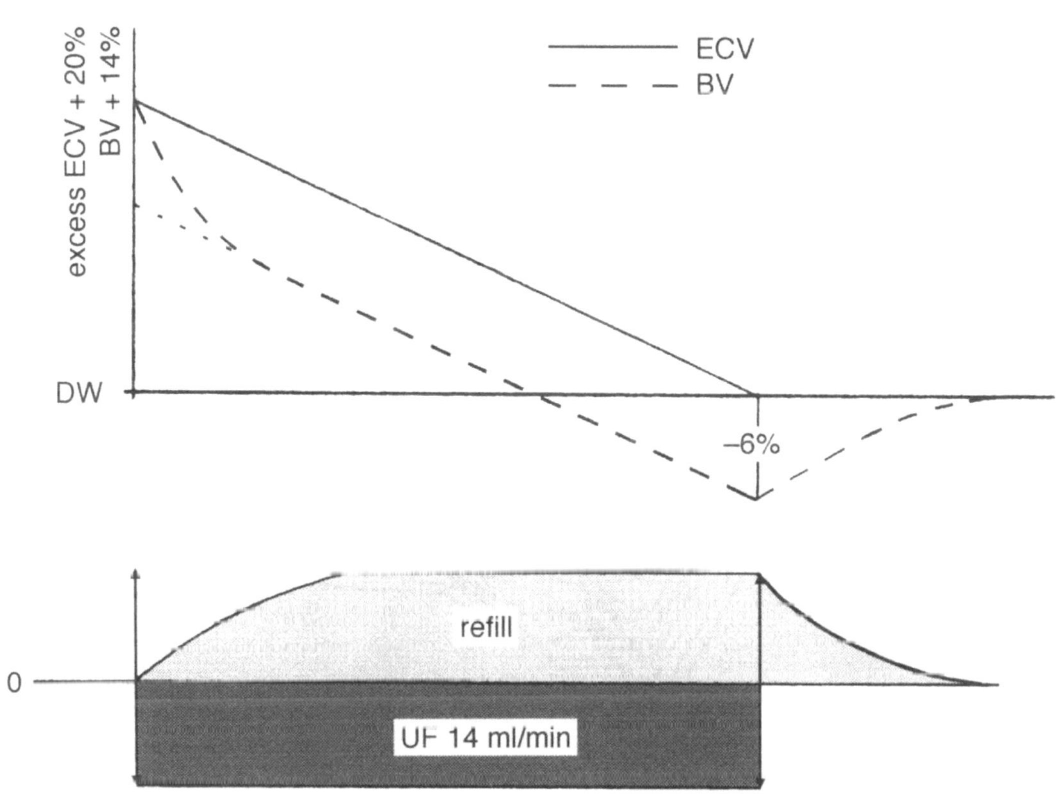

Figure 6.3 Schematic presentation of a patient with extracellular fluid excess of 3.4 L, which is removed by ultrafiltration of 14 ml/min during four hours. Because the refill process lags behind, the blood volume (BV) decreases more rapidly than the ECV. When ultrafiltration is stopped and dry weight has been reached, the blood volume is 6% below the normal value and recovers during the following hour.

capillary to the interstitium or may even reverse it, while the lymph flow will continue to transport fluid back to the vascular compartment. During strong overhydration the compliance of the interstitial space is very large, which means that decrease in its volume will hardly affect the interstitial hydrostatic pressure. However, when normal hydration is approached its compliance decreases and volume reduction will cause the interstitial hydrostatic pressure to drop. This will reduce both the net ultrafiltration pressure and the lymph flow. As a result the rate of refill will slow down.

Therefore the rate of refilling is highly dependent on the *degree of overhydration*. This is illustrated in Figure 6.4 showing that very different changes in BV can be observed during and following a fixed UF volume. Patients with little overhydration showed much more decrease in BV as a result of insufficient refill. The refill continued after UF was stopped. The final blood volume is lower than the initial, but still higher than the value at the end of the UF period. In contrast, severely overhydrated patients showed only a small decrease in blood volume and due to rapid refill their BV finally rose nearly to pretreatment level. This illustrates (as also shown in Figure 3.3) that overhydration not only increases the rate of refill, but also influences the relation between BV and ECV in the steady state. Apart from the hydrostatic and oncotic pressure gradients, the rate of fluid transfer

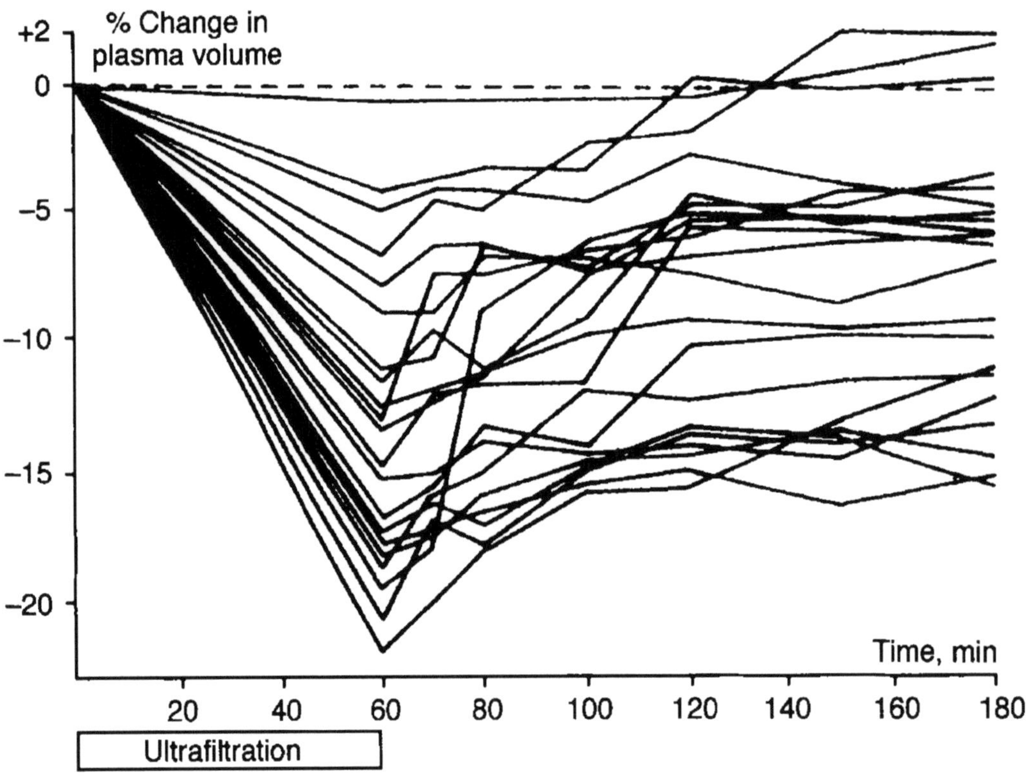

Figure 6.4 Changes in plasma volume after 2 L ultrafiltration. Patients with the largest decrease have the smallest ECV excess (from Koomans et al. 1984, with permission).

at the capillary level is dependent on the ultrafiltration coefficient (Kf), which varies among different tissues. Schneditz calculated the whole body Kf during UF at 5.6 (min 3.2, max 8.0) ml/min mmHg per 50 kg lean body mass (ref. Ch. 3). There are no findings suggesting a change in Kf in dialysis patients. Because the refill fluid also contains some protein (+7 g/L) it is even possible that the final BV may be somewhat higher than the initial BV.

Thus it is during correction of slight overhydration that large changes in BV and therefore hypotensive episodes can be expected. However, complete correction is crucial to achieving a situation where fluid overload does not exist and to preventing hypertension and dilatation of the heart.

From these considerations it is clear that there will always be an overshoot of BV decrease at the end of a dialysis session unless UF is discontinued well before. This overshoot will be proportional to the rate of UF, which is determined by the magnitude of the volume excess and the time available for removal (Figure 6.5). In order to minimize this unwanted effect, it is logical to ultrafiltrate rapidly during the first hour in order to activate the refill process and taper off as soon as normal BV is reached, because the *rate* of BV decrease is probably less important than its absolute decrease for DH to occur. Recently, on-line blood volume monitoring devices have become available based on changes in hematocrit or plasma density. These devices enable visualization of the principles discussed in this chapter and facilitate adaptation of UF schedules. In addition microcomputer software is being developed to modulate UF rate, Na and bicarbonate concentration. The practical usefulness of the latter may be limited, because effects of Na concentration are negligible when compared to the much larger benefits of modulating UF rate alone. Already providers offer possibilities to store up to 18 individual profiles. It is doubtful whether such abundance is really needed. These developments show a laudable revival of interest in volume regulation, but to derive maximal benefit from them the understanding of pathophysiological principles remains necessary.

The dialysis procedure

Of particular interest are the biochemical and other changes induced by the dialysis procedure.

Urea

Urea constitutes the bulk of metabolic products that have to be removed. As urea can pass through cell membranes it is not counted as an osmotically active material. But when the urea level decreases rapidly during HD, it takes some time for the intracellular urea to diffuse out of the cells to the ECV and as long as this process is not completed there exists an *osmotic*

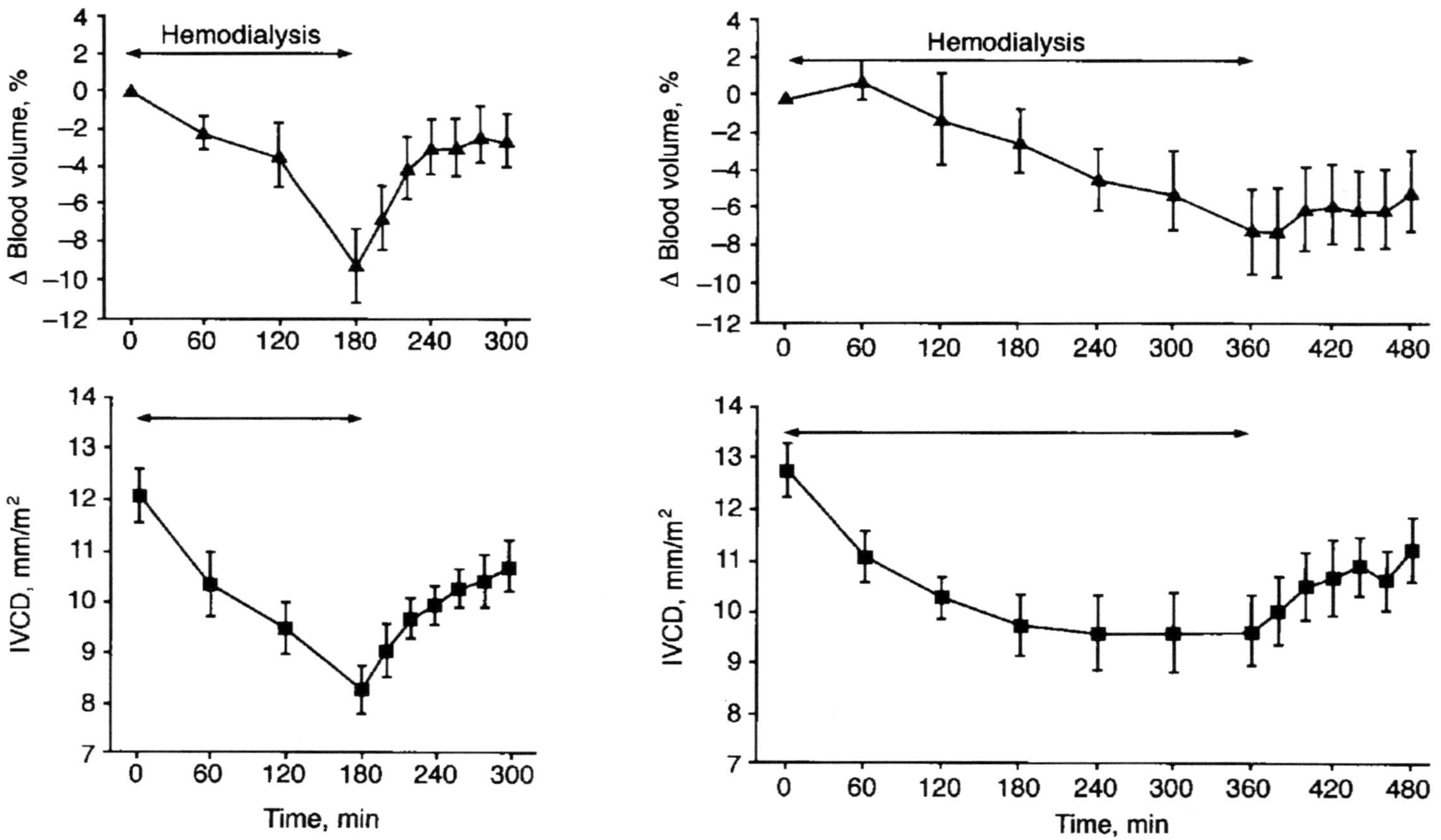

Figure 6.5 Changes in blood volume and inferior vena Cava diameter (IVCD) in a group of patients with 3 hour (left) and a group with 6 hour (right) dialysis. Short dialysis causes much more 'overshoot' (from Katzarski et al. 1997, with permission).

gradient over the cell membrane. Thus urea is *temporarily osmotically active* and attracts water from the interstitial fluid into the cells. This fluid shift during the first dialysis hours is followed by a gradual backflow while the excess urea leaves the cells. The rise in urea (rebound) of 15–20% after a dialysis session indicates that considerable fluid shift must also occur at that time. This refill of the ECV from the cells is added to the plasma refill from the ECV.

Sodium

Sodium and its accompaning anions are nearly exclusively responsible for the osmolarity of the extracellular fluid. Small changes in their concentration result in relatively large fluid shifts from or to the cells, because the intracellular volume is larger. Theoretically a 1% decrease in Na concentration would cause a decrease in ECV of $\pm$0.5 L in a normal man. Conversely use of a dialysis solution with a slightly higher Na concentration than in the patient's blood will attract fluid from the cells and increase the ECV and BV. This effect can be used to counterbalance the action of urea (Figure 6.6). Some authors have advised low-sodium dialysate to decrease hypervolemia, while others have suggested high-sodium dialysate to prevent dialysis hypotension. It is evident that these aims are conflicting: what is good for one is not good for the other. Currently, normal Na concentrations are advocated. There are indications that the increase in Na concentra-

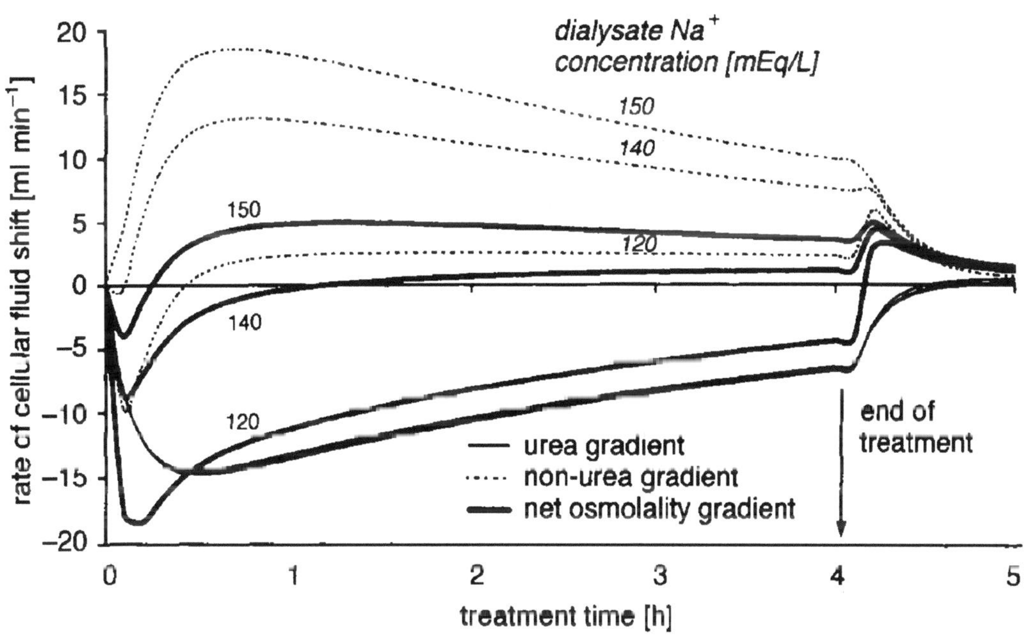

Figure 6.6 Computer simulation of changes in urea and non-urea (in fact NaCl) gradient and fluid shifts during dialysis with hypertonic (150) normotonic (140) and hypotonic (120) Na concentration in dialysate (courtesy of Dr Akcahüseyin (Akahüseyin et al. 2000)).

tion (or osmolality) increases contractility of smooth muscle cells and thus may enhance refill by lowering capillary pressure. These findings await confirmation.

Acetate

For technical reasons acetate has been used instead of bicarbonate in dialysis fluid. Ultimately this would correct interdialytic acidosis equally well because it is metabolized to bicarbonate in the body. However, acetate has several disadvantages. Some patients do not efficiently metabolize acetate, others do not tolerate acetate. Moreover acetate corrects acidosis less completely than does bicarbonate. The main disadvantage of acetate dialysis is that it increases the tendency to DH, because it lowers peripheral resistance. This favors a decrease in BP and causes a decrease in blood flow (pre-load) to the heart. In addition this peripheral vasodilatation may impair plasma refill.

Calcium

With conventional composition of dialysis fluid there is a net positive Ca balance and an increase in Ca blood levels. This has a positive inotropic effect on the heart. Ca infusion has been shown to increase contractility, cardiac output and blood pressure (Figure 6.7).

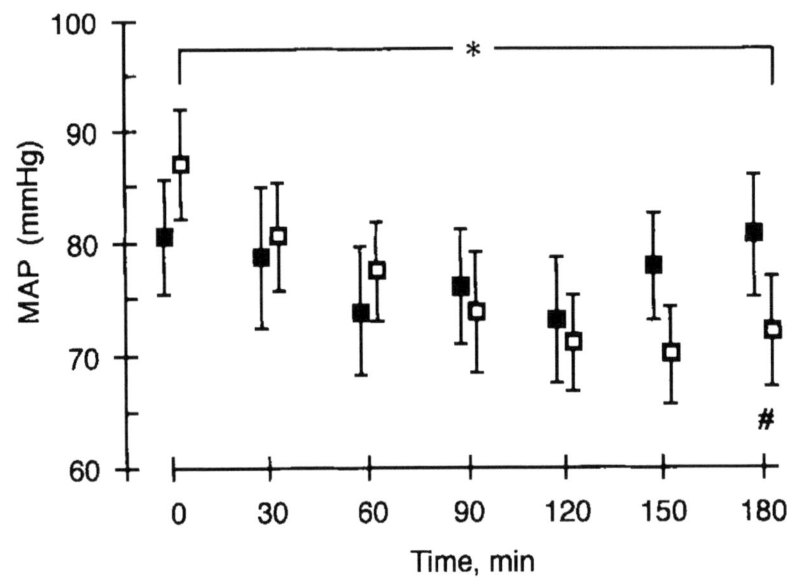

Figure 6.7 Mean arterial pressure (MAP) during dialysis and UF with low Ca (open squares) and high Ca (closed squares) dialysate (from van der Sande et al. 1998, with permission).

Potassium

The bulk of K consumed with the food accumulates in the body and has to be removed during dialysis sessions. This causes a steep drop in K blood levels from supernormal to slightly below normal. This can cause arrhythmias (monitoring during dialysis revealed very frequent ventricular extrasystoles), which could be prevented by lowering potassium levels more slowly. When a patient is digitalized, signs of digitalis toxicity may be precipitated.

Body temperature

During HD an increase in core body temperature occurs, the reason for which has not been completely elucidated. This probably has some hypotensive effect by preventing vasodilation. Anyhow it has been shown that lowering the dialysate temperature has a favorable effect on DH, presumably by sympathetic activation.

The dialysis membrane

It is well known that during dialysis certain reactions take place at the surface of the membrane. There is activation of complement and adhesion of thrombocytes and leukocytes but this does not last beyond the first hour. Such factors have been implicated in the pathogenesis of DH, but no proof has been provided. Indeed one center which continued to use the original cuprophane membranes also reported the lowest incidence of DH (Chazot et al. 1999). The search of more 'biocompatible' membranes is of course welcomed and promoted by the industry. Ironically, one of these new products, AN-69 polyacrilonytril membranes, causes elevated bradykinin levels. While these are most of the time symptomless, they occasionally give rise to anaphylactic reactions. These reactions are provoked by the use of converting enzyme inhibitors, which inhibit bradykinin breakdown (Verresen et al. 1994).

Other factors

The removal of vasoactive substances and hormones during dialysis has been suggested, but there is no proof that this is of any clinical importance. That isolated ultrafiltration is better tolerated than hemodialysis can be attributed mainly to the fact that during isolated UF changes in acetate, urea and body temperature do not occur. As shown in Figure 2.4, eating during dialysis increases hypotension.

The 'uremic state'

In healthy persons acute hypovolemia induces certain adaptations. These probably also happen in dialysis patients but their condition differs from normal in that they start from relative hypervolemia. The large individual variability and the identification of subsets of patients who are particularly prone to DH has led to considerable research into factors that may enhance it.

The veins contain the largest fraction (60%) of the blood and are the most compliant part of the intravascular system. It is uncertain whether active venous constriction occurs in man. Yet a passive decrease in regional blood flow as a result of increased arteriolar resistance causes a shift from the venous compartment towards the heart (de Jager-Krogh phenomenon). This happens particularly in the splanchnic and cutaneous vascular beds. A central shift was also reported during dialysis but not with acetate dialysis. The increase in body temperature may also favour venous pooling. Kooman et al. found decreased venous compliance but only in hypertensive HD patients. They also noticed reduced arteriolar and venous constriction during hemodialysis. Both abnormalities may contribute to DH.

During hypovolemia, increased peripheral resistance occurs which prevents BP from falling and increases venous return as mentioned above. The decreased skin blood flow may be responsible for the rise in body temperature. Arteriosclerosis, which is frequent in dialysis patients and causes decreased arterial compliance, may interfere with this mechanism.

Cardiac functions

Bezold–Jarish reflex

The role of the heart in maintaining circulation and BP in the face of decreasing blood volume is relatively minor. After all, the heart cannot do more than pump the blood that is presented to it. In general there is a stable cardiac output and stroke volume and some increase in pulse rate due to increased sympathetic outflow. The decrease in venous return eventually results in insufficient filling of the heart. At that moment a collapse occurs with sudden decrease in sympathetic activity, bradycardia and 'paradoxical' decreases in peripheral resistance and increase in cardiac output. Abolition of the bradycardia with atropine does not alleviate the hypotension. In the tachycardic type of collapse there is also a decrease in peripheral resistance with increased cardiac output. This suggests that there may not be a fundamental difference between the two types of DH. A similar acute vasovagal reaction can be provoked in normal persons by passive tilting or lower body negative pressure application and is known as the Bezold–Jarish reflex. It is the result of forceful contraction of an empty left ventricle. The nature of a neural reflex as cause of DH is also supported by the rapidity with which it can be reversed by small amounts of volume replacement.

Left ventricular hypertrophy

The Bezold–Jarish reflex is more likely to occur in patients with left ventricular hypertrophy (LVH) and diastolic function impairment ('stiff' ventricle wall), as well as any condition that impairs ventricular filling like tricuspid regurgitation. Because LVH is very frequent in dialysis patients, this appears to be one of the most important factors promoting DH (Figure 6.8). As will be discussed in Chapter 8 the resulting decreased compliance (steeper pressure/volume curve, see Figure 8.5), decreases the tolerance of these patients to both hypo- and hypervolemia. Therefore the presence of LVH will make achievement and maintenance of dry weight more difficult and may indirectly contribute to continuing hypertension and further cardiac damage.

Autonomic nervous system

Many investigators have tried to identify disturbances of baroreceptor reflex function or autonomic impairment to explain why some patients are hypotension prone, but no conclusive evidence has emerged. While it is known that autonomic functions are diminished in diabetic and elderly patients, most hypotension-prone patients have a normal BP reaction on tilting. Likewise, studies on plasma catecholamine levels have failed to show consistent abnormalities in dialysis patients.

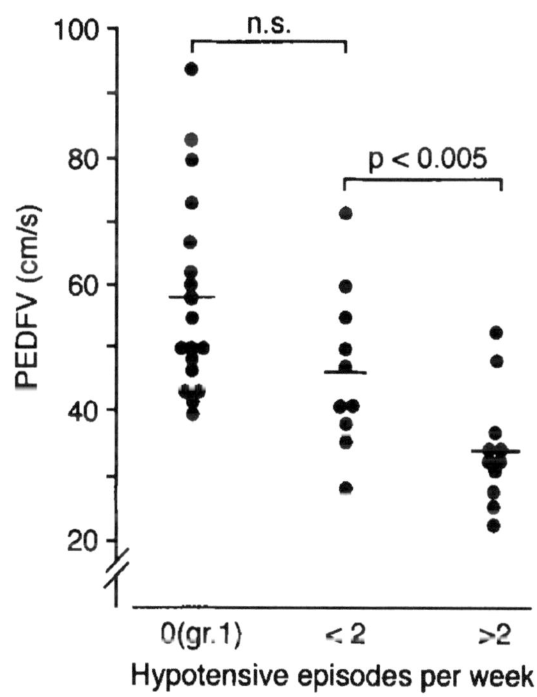

Figure 6.8 Peak velocity of early diastolic filling (PEDFV), a measure of ventricular compliance, in patients with and without hypotensive episodes. Low PEDFV indicates left ventricular hypertrophy (from Ruffmann et al. 1990, with permission).

Renin–angiotensin system

Although the renin–angiotensin system is *hyporeactive* in patients with renal insufficiency, the normal blood pressure response to upright posture of anephric patients argues against a major role of this system in BP adaptation to hypovolemia.

Conclusion

DH may be viewed as a normal physiologic reaction on an unphysiological intervention. The main way to prevent it is to minimize interdialytic weight gain or prolong dialysis time to withdraw the fluid excess more smoothly. 'Overshoot' of BP drop will be decreased by these measures but not completely abolished. To minimize it, dialysis profiling is helpful. This should be aimed at rapid ultrafiltration in the first part of the dialysis session until the desired BV is reached and then tapering it off to keep it at that level. Modulating the dialysate Na level can prevent the initial urea-induced fluid shift, but may be less important than modulating UF rate. The use of BV monitoring devices facilitates this procedure. Additional measures are avoiding acetate dialysis and lowering the dialysate temperature. It is often stated that antihypertensive drugs should be suspended before a dialysis session in order to prevent DH, but the effect of this measure has never been documented. Because the use of antihypertensive drugs makes its virtually impossible to reach dry weight and adapt to a new volume state, these should therefore be suspended altogether during the process of 'probing for dry weight' to allow the BP to adapt to the new volume state. The occurrence of DH is no proof that 'dry weight' has been achieved and can even be observed in the presence of edema. While it may indicate that the goal has been reached, the occurrence of DH is more often the cause of *not* reaching the desired dry weight! The various parameters listed in Chapter 2 are very helpful, but in the large majority of the patients, the ultimate criteria that dry weight has been reached is a normal blood pressure. The time necessary to reach that goal makes it a difficult one to handle.

4 SUSTAINED CHRONIC HYPOTENSION

In contrast to the majority of dialysis patients who are constantly threatened by hypertension, some patients suffer from persistent low blood pressure (systolic pressure lower than 100 mmHg) also between dialysis sessions. When patients with severe dilated cardiomyopathy are excluded, there remains a group in whom the heart is apparently normal and who are not hypovolemic either. Their blood pressure does not increase with volume loading and they have no postural hypotension. In general they are among the long-term dialysis survivors (Figure 6.9).

Hemodynamic studies did not reveal differences in cardiac output or blood volume between hypotensive and normotensive patients. It has been said that these patients easily develop pulmonary congestion upon volume expansion but unfortunately no detailed documentation is available on this important issue. It is clear, however, that the response of their vasculature to vasoconstrictive stimuli is diminished. In some hypotensive patients, high plasma levels of adrenaline, blunted response to phenylephrine infusion and decreased platelet adrenoceptor density were found. Other studies reported elevated renin, angiotensin and aldosteron levels and reduced response to angiotensin infusion, while platelet A2 receptors were reduced compared to normotensive patients. A recent report (Esforzado et al. 1997) found both increased cathecolamines and plasma renin activity but there was an inverse correlation between plasma adrenaline and angiotensin II levels.

It thus appears that the two main vasoconstrictive systems (sympathetic and renin–angiotensin) are activated in a variable manner, probably as a result of *decreased vascular responsiveness*. The reason for the imbalance of the vasoregulatory systems may be increased synthesis of the two endothelin-derived vasodilators: nitric oxide and prostacyclin. Interestingly, this decreased responsiveness seems to be a general feature of long-term dialysis. It may explain the observations that in some dialysis patients' plasma renin

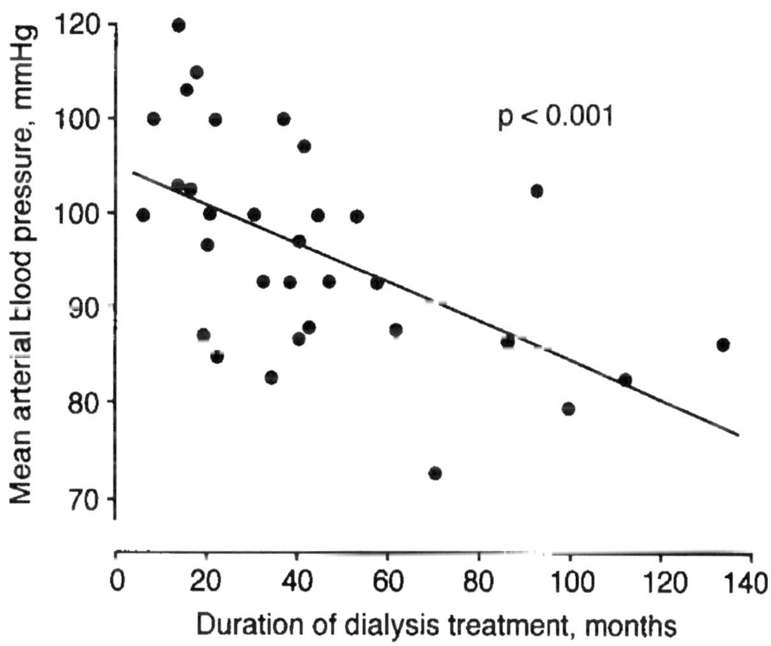

Figure 6.9 Correlation between duration of hemodialysis treatment and mean arterial pressure in 32 patients from one center (from Daul et al. 1987, with permission).

and cathecholamines are elevated but do not correlate with blood pressure. More investigation is needed in this field.

Summary

- Dialysis hypotension is the result of unphysiological, rapid removal of body fluids by ultrafiltration.
- The more weight gain between two sessions and the shorter the dialysis time, the more DH will occur.
- Neither muscle cramps nor DH are proof that 'dry weight' has been reached.
- The mechanism of sudden collapse appears to be a due to reflex-inhibition of sympathetic drive, originating from insufficient filling of the left ventricle.
- Left ventricular hypertrophy sensitizes patients to this reflex.
- The most important factor causing DH is the delay in plasma refill, which is more pronounced when ECV approaches normal levels. Because refill continues after stopping UF, it is almost essential to create a temporal hypovolemia if one ultimately wants to reach normovolemia.
- The dialysis procedure itself causes biochemical and other alterations which favor DH: changes in effective osmolality due to rapid decrease in urea level, acetate, drop in potassium level, rise in body temperature. Except for occasional anaphylactoid reactions the dialysis membrane has no influence.
- ECV refill by urea rebound and plasma refill imply that measurement of circulatory parameters immediately after dialysis causes considerable underestimation of the final blood volume.
- Profiling UF is more helpful than profiling sodium, but the best way to prevent DH is salt restriction and prolongation of dialysis sessions.
- Other measures to prevent DH include stopping hypertensive drugs, using bicarbonate instead of acetate, avoiding eating during dialysis and lowering dialysate temperature.
- Chronic interdialytic hypotension without orthostatic hypotension is a completely different condition. It is seen mainly in patients who have been on dialysis for long periods. Its pathogenesis is thought to be insensitivity of the vasculature to normal vasoconstrictive stimuli.

Bibliography

Akahüseyin E, Nette RW, Vincent HH et al. A simulation study on the intercompartimental fluid shifts during hemodialysis. ASAIO Journal. 2000;46:81–94.

Barnas MGW, Boer WH, Schelven LJ et al. Heart rate variability during dialysis hypotension: confirmation on Bezold–Jarish-like reflex. Kidney Int. 1999;55: 2602.

Daul AE, Wang XL, Michel MC. Arterial hypotension in dialysis patients. Kidney Int. 1987;32:728–35.

Daugirdas JT. Dialysis hypotension: a hemodynamic analysis. Kidney Int. 1991; 39:233–46.

Esforzado N, Cases A, Bono M et al. Vasoactive hormones in uremic patients with chronic hypotension. Nephrol Dial Transplant. 1997;12:321–4.

Katzarski KS, Nisell J, Randmaa I et al. Critical evaluation of ultrasound measurement of inferior vena cava diameter in assessing dry weight in normotensive and hypertensive hemodialysis patients. Am J Kidney Dis. 1997;30:459–65.

Kooman JP, Wijnen JAG, Draayer P et al. Compliance and reactivity of the peripheral venous system in chronic intermittent haemodialysis. Kidney Int. 1992;41:1041–8.

Koomans HA, Geers AB, Dorhout Mees EJ. Plasma volume recovery after ultrafiltration in patients with chronic renal failure. Kidney Int. 1984;26:848–54.

Moore TJ, Lazarus JM, Hakim RM. Reduced angiotensin receptors and pressor responses in hypotensive hemodialysis patients. Kidney Int. 1989;36:696–701.

Ruffmann K, Mandelbauam A, Bommer J et al. Doppler echocardiographic findings in dialysis patients. Nephrol Dial Transplant. 1990;5:426–31.

van der Sande FM, Cheriex EC, van Kuik WHM et al. Effect of dialysate calcium concentrations on intradialytic blood pressure course in cardiac-compromised patients. Am J Kidney Dis. 1998;32:125–31.

Santoro A, Manchini E, Spongano M et al. A haemodynamic study of hypotension during haemodialysis. Nephrol Dial Transplant. 1990;(Suppl. 1):147–53.

Verresen L, Fink E, Lemke H et al. Bradykinin is a mediator of anaphylactoid reactions during hemodiaysis with AN 69 membranes. Kidney Int. 1994;45:1497–503.

Wizemann V, Soetanto R, Thormann J et al. Effects of acetate on left ventricular function in hemodialysis patients. Nephron. 1993;64:101–05.

7

Heart disease in dialysis patients

1 GENERAL CONSIDERATIONS: RISK FACTORS

Natural history

Cardiac disease is the major cause of death in dialysis patients, accounting for half of the total mortality. Clinical manifestations (morbidity of cardiac disease) are equally high. When routinely assessed by echocardiography, the proportion of patients with abnormal dimensions of cardiac compartments is still higher. It should be remarked that this also applies to patients with chronic renal disease. In other words the same pathogenetic mechanisms are present before the start of dialysis treatment. Many patients entering dialysis programs have severe damage already and the complications seen during HD treatment are the result of an ongoing process. Unfortunately, some authors consider it as inexorable fate and speak about the *natural history* of cardiac disease in dialysis patients. This suggests that the development is the result of some *intrinsic* cardiac process, while in reality its course is mainly determined by *extrinsic* factors, i.e. the way of treatment. Dialysis provides a unique opportunity to correct some of these pathogenetic mechanisms and thus slow down, improve, or even cure complications, which once were considered inevitable.

Pathogenesis

Some causes of heart disease are the same as in patients without renal disease: hypertension and atherosclerosis. But there is one all-important difference: *volume overload.* While the failing heart may induce normal kidneys to retain fluid, in HD patients failing kidneys cause primary volume expansion which then damages the heart. The heart can adapt more easily to increased afterload (pressure) than to increased preload (volume). Acute renal failure may even cause heart failure and pulmonary edema in a patient with a normal heart. In 1960 Eichna wrote: "Did the heart really fail? It is hard to see how the heart by improving any of its functions could relieve overfilling". This simple logic is often not taken into account in discussions on this subject. However, the absence of normal volume regulation in terminal renal failure completely upsets all aspects of heart disease in dialysis patients and presents problems with which neither the neprologist nor the cardiologist is familiar.

Prevalence of heart disease and risk factors

Several large studies have documented that cardiovascular mortality is about 9% per year and 10–20 times higher than in the general population. Among dialysis patients in the USA and Canada the prevalence of coronary artery disease is 40% and that of clinically manifest congestive heart failure also 40%. Approximately one-half of cardiac deaths are attributed to cardiac arrest. The relative contribution of arrhythmias is not known.

In many studies sophisticated statistical analysis have been applied to identify *risk factors* and to calculate how much they independently contribute to morbidity and mortality. While such an approach is useful to draw attention once more to these problems, it is of limited value because much depends on the way in which such a group of dialysis patients is treated. For instance in centers where good volume control is applied, congestive heart failure is practically never encountered. In such centers the level of physical activity is higher and the prevalence of hypertension and cardiac dilatation much lower. Neither is much insight gained by stressing that there is 'no evidence yet that interventions for risk factors produce any clinical benefit' (Parfrey et al. 1996) when no studies concerning modification of risk factors are available. Instead of trying to disentangle these interrelated factors we will emphasize the possibilities to influence them. Details of the various cardiological abnormalities will be discussed in the respective sections of Chapter 8.

2 METHODS OF INVESTIGATION

Clinical examination

The setting of hemodialysis treatment does not facilitate classic physical examination, which therefore should preferably be performed on a non-dialysis day. While the absence of *edema* does not exclude overfilling, its presence is of course an important finding. The same applies to *venous pressure elevation* when evidenced by distended neck veins. *Cardiac murmurs* and *friction rubs* can only be detected by auscultation. The dialysis doctor can better evaluate *excessive fistula blood flow* on such a consultation and collect anamnestic information which may not be registered in the busy everyday routine of the dialysis room. Of course this should be supplemented by other techniques.

Chest X ray

A simple chest X-ray is very useful in detecting cardiac abnormalities and is indispensable for evaluating the lungs. Most informative is the overall

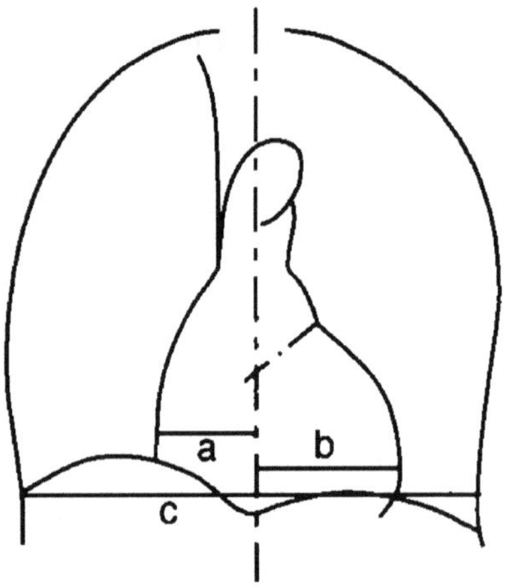

$$\text{Cardiothoracic index (CTi)} = \frac{a+b}{c}$$

Figure 7.1 Schematic presentation of frontal chest X-ray. (a) largest horizontal distance from mid-line to right heart border; (b) idem to left heart border; (c) thorax diameter from inner side of ribs at level of left diaphragm.

dimension of the heart which is expressed as the cardiothoracic index (CTi). This is the largest width of the heart divided by the largest inner diameter of the thoracic cage (Figure 7.1). Despite a number of inaccuracies, related to the structure of the thorax, the position of the heart, the level of inspiration and the phase of cardiac contraction, it gives invaluable information, in particular for follow-up of the same patient. The upper limit of normal is often given as 0.50, but in my experience this is too high. Depending on the individual, normal values vary between 0.36 and 0.46. If the CTi is increased, this may be for several reasons which have to be differentiated with an echocardiogram. Muscular hypertrophy can give some enlargement, but very marked increases well over 0.50 are nearly always caused by cardiac dilatation or pericardial effusion.

The importance of changes in hydration of the patient is illustrated by the fact that the CTi may acutely decrease by 0.5–1 cm when 3 kg excess is ultrafiltrated during a dialysis session. The accuracy of the CTi may be improved by better standardization, but this has not been attempted to my knowledge, and comparisons with the much more accurate echocardiography are scarce.

Electrocardiography

This classic method is of course indispensable to investigate arrhythmia's and myocardial ischemia and infarction. Left ventricular hypertrophy (LVH) may be detected also, but quantitative assessment needs the application of echocardiography. Contrary to expectation the ECG is very often normal in 'uremic' pericarditis.

Echocardiography

Echocardiography is the standard reference method, which provides quantitative information both on the structure and on the function of the heart. Being non-invasive it can easily be repeated in the same patient. Given the importance of these problems and the fact that the information cannot be obtained by other means, every dialysis center should have easy access to (or better, operate itself) an echocardiograph. There are several techniques (modes) as depicted in Figure 7.2.

M-mode (motion mode)

This displays the ultrasound reflections on a paper moving at constant speed and thus gives a single-dimension–time image.

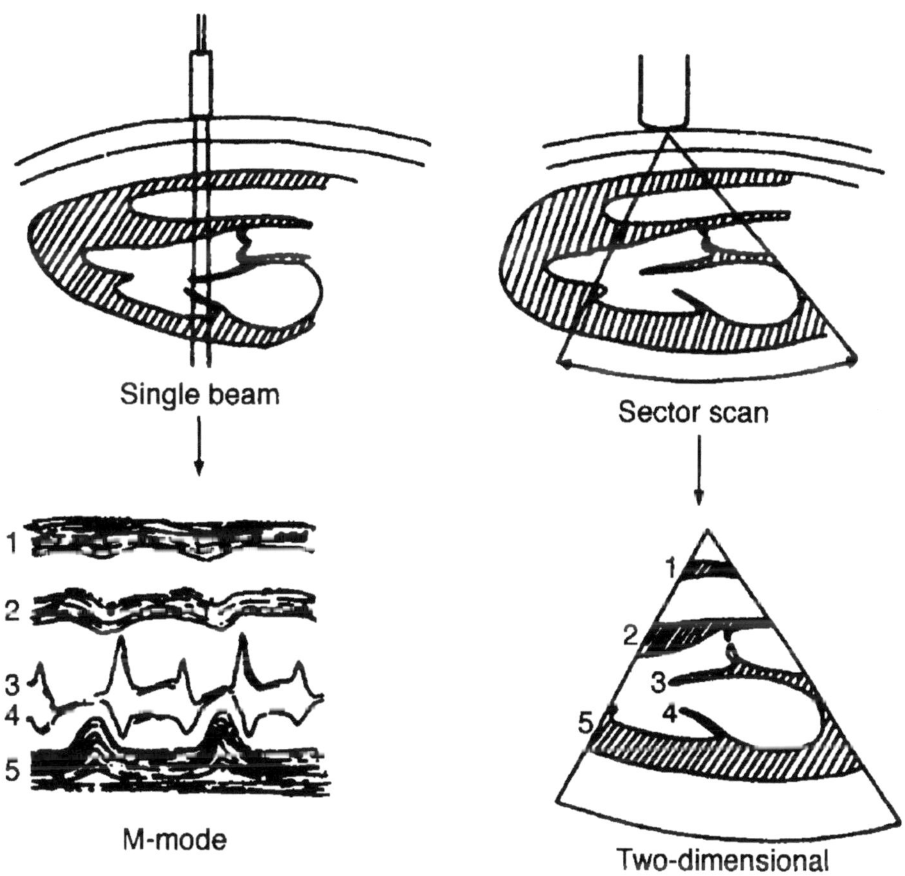

Figure 7.2 Schematic presentation of echocardiographic techniques.

Two-dimensional ('real time')

This gives a two-dimensional cut of a segment of the heart that can be 'frozen' or videotaped.

Both methods are useful for recording thickness of compartment walls, effusion layers and cavity diameters and volumes. From diastolic (D) and systolic (S) ventricle volumes (V), stroke volume and ejection fraction (EF) can be calculated as follows:

$$\text{Stroke volume} = DV - SV$$

$$EF = \text{Stroke volume}/DV \times 100$$

Furthermore *systolic functions* of the left ventricle (LV) can be derived: fractional fibre shortening (FS) and velocity of circumferential shortening (Vcf). Some normal values are given in Table 7.1.

Doppler ultrasound

This method compares the frequency of the transmitted with that of the received ultrasound, reflected off by moving blood cells. Cells moving towards the transducer cause a higher frequency than those moving away. There are several modalities, among them *colour Doppler.* The Doppler method can measure blood velocity and establish site and direction of abnormal blood flow, such as valvular stenosis and regurgitation. If tricuspid regurgitation is present, the *pulmonary artery pressure* can be estimated. Consequently the Doppler method has obviated the need for cardiac catheterization in many cases.

Table 7.1 Normal echocardiographic values in adults

Dimension (cm)	Mean	Ranges
LVDd	4.6	3.6–5.4
LVDs	2.9	2.0–3.9
LAD	2.9	1.9–4.0
RVDd	1.6	0.8–2.4
LVPWd	0.9	0.7–1.1
IVd	0.9	0.7–1.2
Functions		
EF	0.7	0.6–0.8
VCf circ/sec	1.4	1.1–1.8
E/A ratio	1.6	1.2–2.0

L left, R right, V ventricle, D diameter, s systolic, d diastolic, PW posterial wall, IVS interventricular septum, EF ejection fraction, VCf velocity of circumferential fiber shortening, E/A ratio of early to late (atrial) phase of ventricular filling.
For other diastolic functions see Figure 7.3.

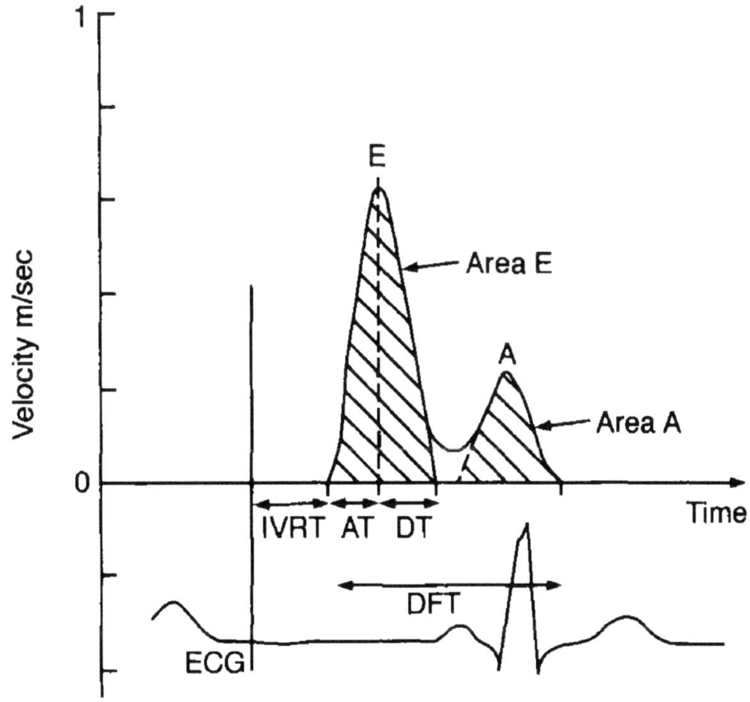

Figure 7.3 Pulsed wave Doppler echo of normal mitral valve and calculation of diastolic indices. A = aortic valve closure, IVRT = isovolumic relaxation time, AT = acceleration time, DT = deceleration time, DFT = total diastolic filling time.

Another important application is evaluation of *diastolic function* of the LV. The flow pattern through the normal mitral valve depends on atrial systolic function and left ventricular stiffness, which is often disturbed when hypertrophy is present. A much-used parameter is the E/A ratio, indicating the ratio of early (E) to late atrial active (A), filling velocity–time integral, as illustrated in Figure 7.3. The early filling is determined by the ventricular *relaxation* which is an active process using energy. Some other derived parameters of diastolic function are also shown in this figure and normal values in Table 7.1.

Interpretation of echocardiographic results

It should be remarked that the accuracy of much echocardiographic estimation is limited. First of all, the method error is ± 2 mm, which means that in measuring small dimensions like wall thickness a systematic error up to 20% is inevitable. Second, the position of the tranducer is critical for good measurements, which requires experience in the echographist. Furthermore some pathophysiological knowledge is necessary to interpret the results. In particular, loading conditions profoundly influence the functional parameters. Due to the very frequently occurring hypervolemia in dialysis patients an increased left ventricular end-diastolic diameter is found. If volume decreases after a period of ultrafiltration, end-diastolic diameter decreases and the shortening fraction (often used as a surrogate for ejection fraction) may decrease, although the intrinsic function of the ventricle remains unchanged. Conversely a decrease in afterload (blood pressure) will cause a decrease in left ventricular systolic diameter resulting in an increased EF and better contractility. If these considerations are not taken into account, such changes may be wrongly attributed to changes in intrinsic functions of the ventricle.

Even more caution is required when interpreting *diastolic function.* The rapid early filling phase of the left ventricle (E) decreases when the compliance of the ventricle wall is decreased, which often results from hypertrophy, infarction or fibrotic changes. Thus the second phase (atrial contraction) compensatory becomes more important resulting in a decreased E/A ratio. However, elevated atrial pressure (caused by hypervolemia) will increase phase E and its decrease during ultrafiltration might erroneously be interpreted as deterioration of ventricular diastolic function (Figure 7.4).

Summary

- Heart disease in chronic renal patients is to a large extent secondary to hypertension and volume expansion.
- The heart can adapt better to chronic increase in pressure than to increase in volume load.

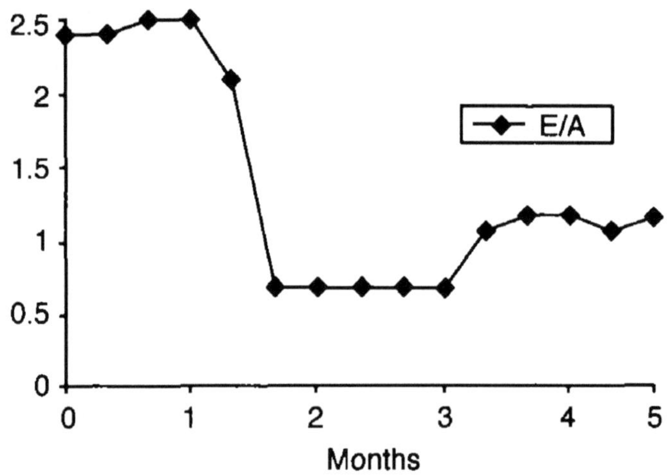

Figure 7.4 Changes in diastolic function during correction of cardiomyopathy. The E/A ratio, representing early to late left venticular filling (normal value 1.6) was initially elevated because of a high left atrial pressure. After improvement it dropped to pathological low values, reflecting the decreased compliance of the hypertrophied left ventricle. With regression of hypertrophy and remodelling of the dilated ventricle wall, E/A ratio rose again to near-normal values. This illustrates the predominant role of *loading conditions* which may obscure intrinsic abnormality of the muscle wall (data from patient described on page 91).

- Dialysis treatment offers an opportunity to correct these abnormalities and favorably influence the course of some cardiac disturbances.
- Regular clinical examination and chest X-ray can give very useful information and should not be neglected but echocardiography and Doppler ultrasound are almost indispensable methods for evaluation and follow-up of many patients.
- While dimensions of cardiac cavities can be easily understood, some understanding of the basic pathophysioloic principles is necessary to interpret functional parameters provided by the echocardiogram.

Bibliography

Blaustein AS, Schmidt G, Foster MC et al. Serial effects on left ventricular load and contractility during hemodialysis. Am Heart J. 1986;111:340–6.

Don C, Burns KD, Levine DZ. Body fluid volume status in hemodialysis patients: the value of the chest radiograph. J Can Ass Radiol. 1990;41:123–6.

Eichna LW. Circulatory congestion and heart failure. Circulation. 1960;22:864–5.

Harnett JD, Murphy B, Collingwood P et al. The reliability and validity of echocardiographic measurements of left ventricular mass index in hemodialysis patients. Nephron. 1993;65:212–14.

Ishida Y, Meisner JS, Tsunoka et al. Left ventricular filling dynamics: influence of left ventricular relaxation and left atrial pressure. Circulation. 1986;74:187–96.

Madsen BR, Allpert MA, Whiting RB et al. Effect of hemodialysis on left ventricular performance. Am J Nephrol. 1984;4:86–91.

Parfrey PS, Folely RN, Harnett JD et al. Outcome and risk factors for left ventricular disorers in chronic uremia. Nephrol Dial Transplant. 1996;11:1277–85.

Tomson CRV. Echocardiographic assessment of systolic function in dialysis patients. Nephrol Dial Transplant. 1990;5:325–33.

Wizemann V, Kramer W. Choice of ESRD strategy according to cardiac status. Kidney Int. 1988;33(Suppl. 24):191–5.

8

Special aspects of dialysis-related heart disease

1 CARDIAC DILATION

As we saw in the preceding pages, volume retention inevitably leads to dilatation of the heart compartments. This first becomes apparent in increases of left atrial, ventricular end diastolic diameters and volumes. Published data reveal that values in the upper range of normal are the rule (London et al. 1993) and frank dilatation very frequent (between 20% and 50% in different series). This fact alone strongly suggests inadequate volume control in a large proportion of the dialysis population. Indeed a direct relationship was found between blood volume and LVDd.

Dilatation of the left atrium is particularly frequent and persistent in dialysis patients. It is clearly related to volume overload because the atrial diameter acutely decreases with ultrafiltration, but also dependent on the condition of the left ventricle. When the compliance of the left ventricle is decreased as a result of muscular hypertrophy, increased atrial pressure is needed to fill it. Thus it may not be possible to normalize atrial dilatation completely by ultrafiltration so long as left ventricular hypertrophy persists.

Other causes of cardiac enlargement are high-flow AV fistulas (Figure 8.1) and anemia (see Chapter 10). However, part of the mechanism involved may still be volume expansion.

Moderate LV dilatation is associated with higher mortality, while patients with strong dilatation and little hypertrophy (high vol./mass ratio) have a particularly bad prognosis (Foley et al. 1995). Although hypervolemia causes hypertension as well as cardiac dilatation, both of which are risk factors, hypervolemia per se is never mentioned as an independent risk factor. One of the reasons may be that parameters of volume retention are not usually recorded. Nevertheless, the fact that volume retention is a very strong risk factor is of prime importance for the treatment of dialysis patients.

2 LEFT VENTRICULAR HYPERTROPHY

Left ventricular hypertrophy is present in more than 60% of ESRD patients. It is *not* an innocuous adaptation, but a strong risk factor. In essential hypertension, no other risk factor approaches LVH in potency and it affects prognosis very unfavorably in dialysis patients as well (Silberberg et al.

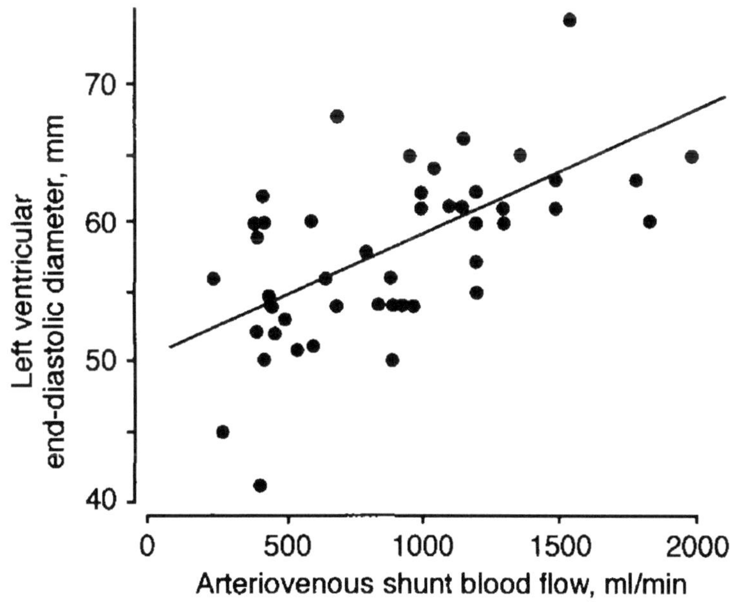

Figure 8.1 Correlation between arteriovenous shunt flow and left ventricular end-diastolic diameter in hemodialysis patients. $R = 0.62$, $P < 0.0001$ (from London et al. 1993, with permission).

1989). Why is LVH so harmful? First of all it is a marker for end-organ damage by long lasting hypertension, among which is coronary artery disease. But increased ventricular muscle mass may itself contribute to coronary risk through increased oxygen demand and impaired endocardial autoregulation. In addition, hypertrophy is associated with increased interstitial fibrosis and decreased capillary density, which probably provide the substrate for malignant arrhytmhia's. As a result, the risk of sudden death and other cardiac events is many times higher with, than without LVH. In addition, LVH is the main cause of diastolic functional disturbances.

Diagnosis

Electrocardiographic changes (high voltage, ST changes) can be seen in severe cases, but are 5–10 times less sensitive than echocardiography. The chest X-ray (cardiothoracic index, CTi) is the least sensitive, because of the large normal variability and other limiting factors. In general a CTi >50% is not due to hypertrophy only, unless it is exceptionally severe. The most sensitive method is echocardiography, which enables us to measure left ventricular mass (LVM) in grams. However, calculation of the LVM is tricky, as it involves subtraction of two volumes. Errors increase when the volume of the heart changes.

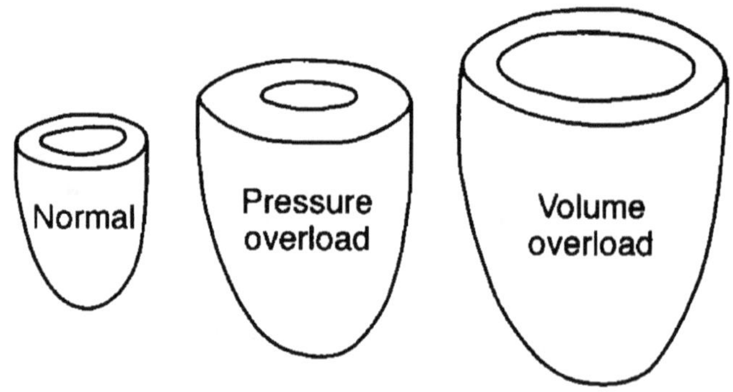

LV wall thickness (mm)	8.2	15.2	10.6
σ_m(10^3 dynes/cm^2)			
Peak Systolic	150	160	175
End Diastolic	17	23	41

Figure 8.2 Types of hypertrophy LV = left ventricle, σ_m = wall stress. Approximate figures, adapted from Grossman 1975. Note that end-diastolic wall stress is strongly elevated in dilated LVH.

There are two types of LVH (Figure 8.2). Pressure overload, (hypertension) causes proliferation of sarcomeres in parallel, resulting in thickening of the myocardium. This is measured at the interventricular septum (IVS) as well as at the posterior wall (PW). The IVS usually increases more than the PW. This *'asymmetric'* hypertrophy was once considered to be pathognomic for certain disease states, including chronic renal failure, but it is probably an *aspecific* phenomenon caused by geometric conditions of the ventricle. When the ventricle does not dilate, the muscle mass/volume ratio increases. This is called 'concentric' hypertrophy.

Volume overload with dilatation of the heart causes proliferation of the sarcomeres in series. To this condition the rather confusing term 'eccentric' hypertrophy is applied. In that situation, both the volume and the muscle mass are increased. While in uncomplicated hypertension and in physiological fitness training the ventricular muscle mass-to-volume ratio is increased, it may remain normal or even decrease when dilatation is present.

It is important to realize how harmful ventricular dilatation is. According to La Place's law, the relation between the radius of the ventricle and the wall thickness determines the wall stress (force per cm of muscle, necessary to eject the blood). For instance, if the diameter increases by 1.4 a nearly threefold increase in muscle mass is required to restore the wall stress, an effect similar to that of an increase in systolic BP by 100 mmHg. In addition it was found that 'excentric' hypertrophy can normalize systolic, but not diastolic wall stress. Because wall stress is one of the factors determining the oxygen demand of the myocardium, pathological increase will worsen symptoms of coronary insufficiency.

Pathogenesis

The factors contributing to the LVH of dialysis patients are the following.

Hypertension

Long periods of insufficiently treated hypertension often precede dialysis treatment and during dialysis normotension is often not achieved.

Fluid retention

Fluid retention causing expansion of the BV is extremely frequent in dialysis patients. But even if left ventricular internal dimensions are sometimes normalized during ultrafiltration, they increase again in the interdialytic interval. This *harmonica effect* is not innocuous, as shown by the relationship between interdialytic weight changes and LVH (London et al. 1993).

Arterial changes

In hypertensive end-stage renal patients the large arteries have larger diameters and decreased distensability as compared to hypertensive patients without renal disease. The decreased elasticity increases the pulsatile work of the heart at the expense of continuous work. (see also Chapter 9). The resulting increase in *pulse pressure* (difference between systolic and diastolic pressure), pulse wave velocity and wave reflections constitute an independent risk factor for LVH (Figure 8.3).

Chronic anemia

One of the hallmarks of renal failure, chronic anemia gives rise to a hyperdynamic circulation in order to satisfy the oxygen demands of the tissues. This is accompanied by dilatation of the left ventricle and atrium. Anemia has been shown to be a strong determinant of LVH, while erythropoietin treatment can cause regression. Some investigations suggest that a low hemoglobin level also causes LVH by itself (see also Chapter 10).

Shunts

Another factor which causes increased volume load is the arterio-venous shunt (AVS). In one study, compression of the shunt caused 0.6 L decrease in cardiac output. Like anemia it results in decreased vascular resistance and increase in venous return, stroke volume and heart rate. The radial artery shunt seldom causes flow rates of more than 10% of cardiac output, but brachial artery shunts may have flow-rates of 1 L/min and more, and

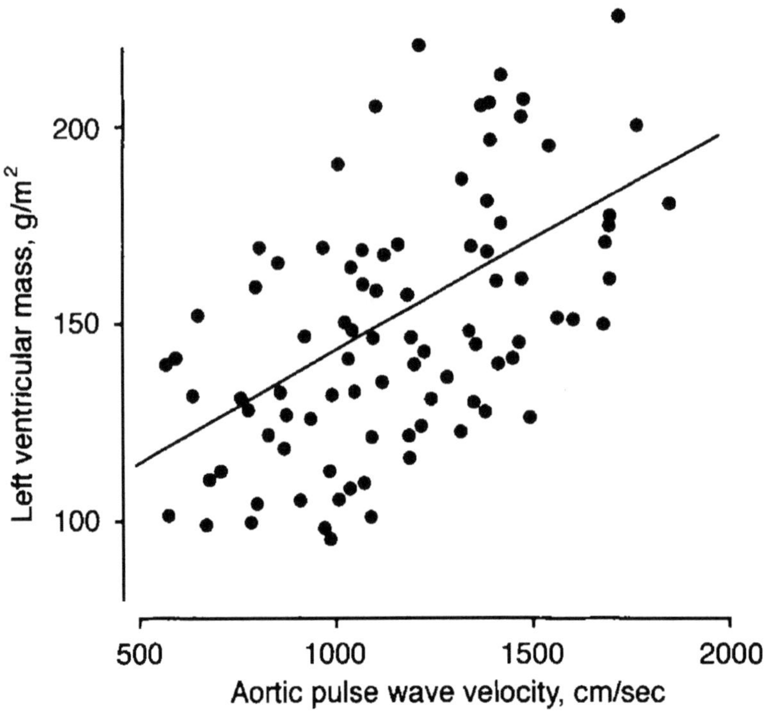

Figure 8.3 Correlation between aortic pulse wave velocity and left ventricular mass in hemodialysis patients $r = 0.52$, $P < 0.001$ (from London et al. 1993 with permission).

should be avoided if possible. Regular control of AVS should be performed by dialysis personnel. Apart from Doppler flow measurement, a test which is easy to perform is manual compression of the shunt. An acute decrease in pulse rate upon this maneuver is a sure sign that the shunt is hemodynamically important, and surgical correction should be considered.

Toxic factors

Uremic patients and experimental animals may show myocardial fibrosis and microvascular alterations which cannot be explained by volume and pressure overload (Amann et al. 1995). Even with excellent control of volume and blood pressure over prolonged periods, LVH persisted and showed no signs of regression in some series.

Other factors

Other factors have been implicated, the most important being secondary hyperparathyroidism. Unequivocal proof of this contention is not available. Calcifications of peripheral arteries, the mitral annulus, and the mitral and aortic valves, and in the myocardium are frequent in dialysis patients and increase with duration of dialysis. Hyperparathyroidism is not the only factor involved, and high phosphate levels by themselves lead also to calcifications. If aortic stenosis develops, this contributes very seriously to LVH.

Prevention and treatment of LVH

Blood pressure and volume correction

In patients with normal renal function, reduction of pressure (hypertension treatment) and volume overload (replacement of deficient valves) can reverse LVH, although some of the histological changes may not regress completely. It can therefore be expected that LVH in dialysis patients will also improve by appropriate treatment. However, most authors failed to achieve regression and they even consider LVH in dialysis patients to be an unavoidable progressive condition. The concern with risk factors and the stress on 'uremic cardiomyopathy' have unfortunately created a fatalistic attitude. Failure to correct hidden volume expansion may at least partially explain the persistence of LVH. This contention is supported by studies on daily home dialysis, which greatly facilitates volume control. While antihypertensive drugs were stopped, a gradual decrease in BP accompanied by a significant decrease in left atrial and ventricular diameters together with regression of LVH were noticed (Buoncristiani et al. 1996). However, this result can also be achieved with conventional dialysis sessions three times a week. A group of 15 hypertensive dialysis patients whose BP was initially lowered by intensified ultrafiltration were followed up for a mean of three years (Özkahya et al. 1998). During this period there was a further decrease in the already improved cardiac dimensions while left ventricular muscle mass showed a marked decrease (Table 8.1).

A striking observation was that BP became progressively easier to control. Probably the decrease in LVH improves cardiac diastolic compliance and, by decreasing the danger of sudden BP drop during UF, facilitates volume control (see Chapter 6). It thus appears that decreasing volume load is at least as important as lowering BP and that these two measures influence each other favorably.

Drug treatment

In sharp contrast to patients with essential hypertension where regression of LVH after various drug treatments has been amply documented, it appears difficult to achieve this result in dialysis patients, despite large-scale use of multiple drugs. Only recently, studies in selected patient groups have reported regression of LVH after drug treatment, but only when the regimen included a converting enzyme inhibitor (CEI). This was accompanied by a decrease in left ventricular diameter, which raises the question whether or not a decrease in volume had also contributed to the result. In one such

Table 8.1 Regression of LVH after persistent volume control

	Time months	BP	CTi (%)	LVdi	LVsi	LVMi
Initial	0	191/109	54	–	–	–
1st echo	2	137/88	48	28.3	18.7	175
2nd echo	16	129/80	45	25.6	17.4	136
3rd echo	37	116/73	43	24.6	15.9	105

Results of severe salt restriction, ultrafiltration and stopping antihypertensive drugs in a group of 15 hypertensive patients who had been on hemodialysis for 8–48 months.
After acceptable blood pressure (BP) was achieved (two months after start of the new regimen) the first echocardiogram was taken and the regimen was continued. Note that, while left ventricular mass index (LVMi) decreased strikingly, there were also modest but significant further decreases in BP, cardiothoracic index (CTi) and left ventricular diastolic (LVdi) and systolic diameter index (LVsi). All changes between first and 3rd echo were highly significant. For simplicity only mean values are given. From Özkahya et al. 1998.

study, blood pressure did not drop immediately after starting the drug, but very slowly decreased during the four years follow up (Figure 8.4). However the decrease in LVH was only *significant* in patients *not* bearing the delayed allele of the angiotensin converting enzyme gene (Canella et al. 1998). The same authors observed that low-dose converting enzyme inhibitor induced regression of LVH without affecting blood pressure in normotensive dialysis patients (in whom left ventricular diameter also decreased). Others found that CEI with high affinity for cardiac converting enzyme, like quinalapril, are more effective. These findings support the concept that not only do these drugs act by lowering blood pressure, but also directly influence remodeling of the cardiac muscle and/or by a similar action on the large arteries increase their compliance and lower the wave reflections. Another explanation would be that renin-lowering drugs somehow facilitate volume control.

Correction of anemia

Many studies have documented regression of LVH after treatment with erythropoetin, but only in patients whose volumes and blood pressure were well controlled. As will be discussed in Chapter 11, the relative ease with which this could be achieved forms one more argument for the importance of volume load in the pathogenesis of LVH.

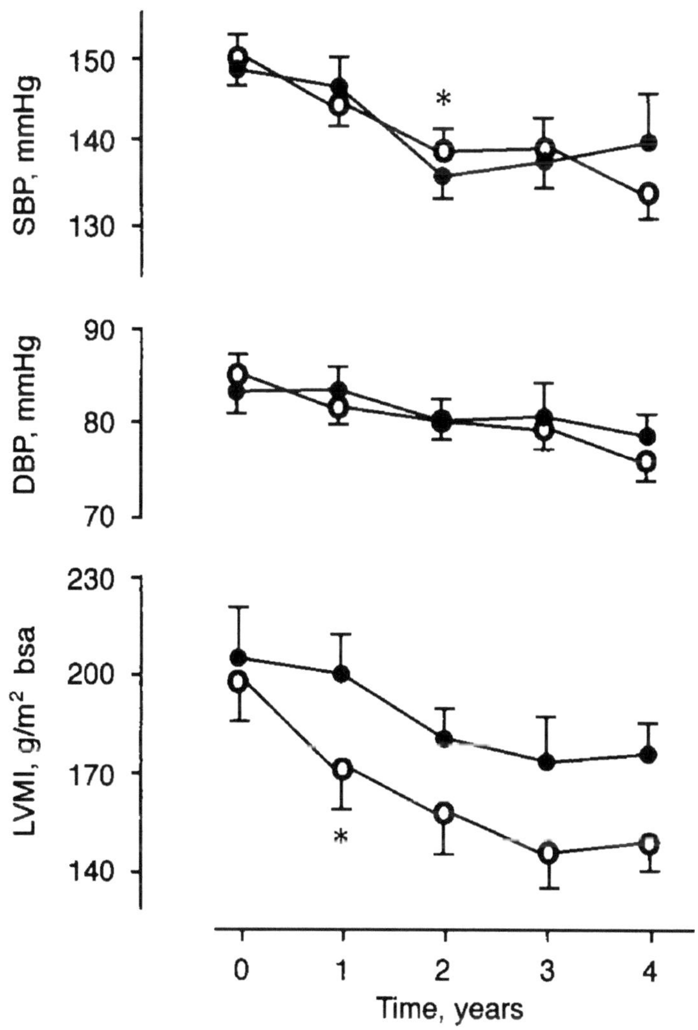

Figure 8.4 Values of 24-hour systolic (S) and diastolic (D) blood pressures (BP) and left ventricular mass indices (LVM) for groups of hypertensive hemodialysed uremics bearing the DD or II/ID.ACE-gene genotype while on antihypertensive therapy with ACE inhibitors (from Canella et al. 1998, with permission).

3 CONGESTIVE HEART FAILURE

Left- or right-sided failure

A cardinal feature of congestive heart failure (CHF) is the presence of circulatory congestion. This congestion involves the venous beds behind the left side of the heart, the right side, or both. Congestion behind the left ventricle causes the dyspnea, orthopnea and pulmonary edema. Venous congestion behind the right ventricle produces characteristically distended veins, enlarged liver and edema. While these two types of congestion often co-exist, the former mostly dominates the clinical picture in dialysis patients. Right-sided congestion becomes manifest later, when the heart is more severely damaged and will be discussed in Dilated cardiomyopathy, below.

When speaking about 'heart failure', reviewers usually mean symptomatic pulmonary congestion. In one such study (Harnett et al. 1995), it was present in 31% of the patients at the start of HD, and recurred in 56%. Of the remaining patients 25% later developed CHF *de novo*. Thus 34% of all patients had at least one episode of CHF during HD treatment! Patients with pulmonary congestion have varying degrees of dilatation and systolic and diastolic dysfunction of the left ventricle. Some of them are hyperkinetic and have normal ejection fractions. As we have seen, that hypervolemia may cause pulmonary congestion even with a normal heart, it is of no use to try to distinguish between intrinsic heart failure and volume overload. Not only are the clinical findings indistinguishable, but hypervolemia is a factor in nearly all cases, and also when the heart is damaged. This is illustrated by the beneficial effect of UF (by hemodialysis or peritoneal dialysis) in patients with severe cardiac failure and normal kidneys.

Clinical presentation

Pulmonary edema characteristically develops acutely in a patient with subclinical congestion, apparently by some change in the subtle balance of 'Starling forces' in the lung. Minor degrees of pulmonary congestion can often be detected on the chest X-ray of HD patients, while modern techniques have revealed increased fluid content of the lungs in the majority of symptomless HD patients (Wallin et al. 1996). Pulmonary edema may give strange pictures, butterfly appearance with cloud-like densities on the chest X-ray Pleural effusions are also involved and may give round shadows ('fading tumors') when localized in the interlobular space.

Pathophysiology

Toxic factors?

The unusual X-ray appearances have been called 'uremic', and are believed to be related to increased permeability of the lung capillaries due to 'uremic toxins'. It was shown recently that this theory is not correct and that there is no pathophysiological difference between lung edema in patients with and without renal failure. There is, however, a most important *etiological* difference: in HD patients; the *primary* cause is fluid retention. While this also causes congestion when the heart is normal, it occurs most of the time in patients with varying degrees of cardiac damage.

Adaptation with time

A very important factor determining the accumulation of fluid in the lungs at any given level of pulmonary capillary pressure is the functional capacity of the lymphatics. In patients with longstanding subclinical congestion, lymphatic capacity increases remarkably (Szidon 1989). Thus, while normally, pulmonary edema may occur at pulmonary capillary pressures of 18 mmHg, it may not occur in adapted patients until it rises well over 25 mmHg. This explains the paradox that symptomatic congestion ('failure') is mainly seen in patients with good left ventricular systolic function.

Diastolic functional impairment

A major factor, which lowers the threshold for pulmonary edema, is disturbed diastolic function resulting from LVH. This function can be summarized as *compliance* of the left ventricle. Decreased compliance means that the curve relating changes in pressure to changes in volume (dP/dV) becomes steeper, as illustrated in Figure 8.5. The impaired relaxation leads to an exaggerated increase in end-diastolic pressure for a given increase in LV end-diastolic volume. As a result increased pulmonary capillary pressure and lung edema develop earlier. Conversely, the decreased compliance

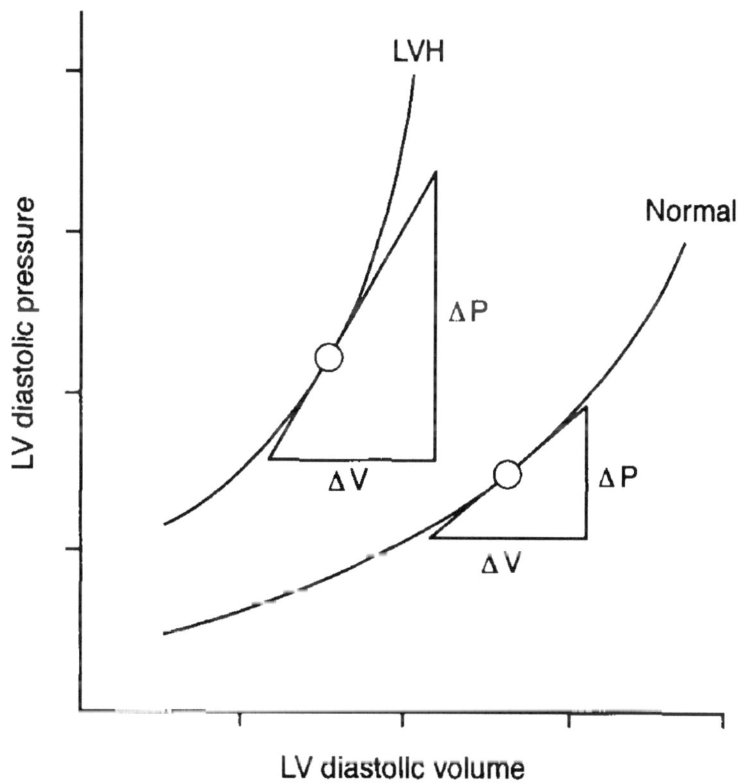

Figure 8.5 Pressure–volume relationship of the left ventricle during diastolic filling. Right: normal heart, Left: heart with left ventricular hypertrophy. The latter curve is shifted upward. That means that more pressure is needed to reach a given diastolic volume. The curve is also steeper: Any increment or decrement of volume (ΔV) is associated with an exaggerated increase or decrease in pressure (ΔP).

Table 8.2 Cardiac effects of 2.9 kg increase in body weight

	Heart vol. (ml/m)^2	LVDP	PAP R	PAP E	MAP R	MAP E	CI (L/min) R	CI (L/min) E
Contr.	409	10	14	28	122	131	6.7	13
Exp.	611	20	26	41	131	109	6.6	11

In this group of "clinically normal" but hypertensive dialysis patients, intracardiac pressures were in the upper normal limits, but after increased volume both LVDP (upper limit 12 mmHg) and PAP (upper limit 15 mmHg) rose to pathological levels. Exercise revealed the loss of reserve and during expansion caused incipient decompensation, shown by the drop in MAP.
Contr. = before weight gain; Exp = during increased weight; R = rest; E = exercise; LVDP = left ventricular end diastolic pressure; PAP = pulmonary artery pressure; MAP = mean arterial pressure (all in mmHg); CI = cardiac index (L/min); Heart vol. and CI given per m^2 body surface area. Data from Golf et al. 1983.

also causes a more rapid decline in pressure when volume (preload) decreases, thus favoring the occurrence of hypotension during UF as well.

A classic paper by Golf (1983) showing the effects of an increase of 2.9 L in ECV in clinically normal HD patients illustrates the principles discussed in this section (Table 8.2). The combined effect of exercise and overhydration caused pulmonary artery and wedge pressures compatible with impending pulmonary edema and revealed a greatly reduced cardiac reserve capacity. The authors concluded that 'it is not unusual to have patients grossly overhydrated for months or years' in dialysis praxis. Incidentally they emphasize the usefulness of individual changes in heart size at chest X-ray as an indicator of volume load.

4 VALVULAR DISEASE

Cardiac murmurs are often heard in dialysis patients and may disappear during treatment. They have been called 'functional' in the past and attributed to anemia or high output state. Systematic use of Doppler echocardiography, however, has brought sound proof that valvular (in particular mitral) regurgitation is indeed frequent. Interestingly, there appears to be a poor correlation between auscultatory and Doppler findings.

Mitral regurgitation

The incidence of mitral regurgitation (MR) varies between 13% and 44% in different reports. It may appear *de novo* during treatment and is associated with a bad prognosis. Two possible etiological factors have been proposed: *calcifications* of the mitral annulus and *dilatation* of the annulus as a result of cardiac dilatation and overhydration.

Calcifications of the annulus (and less often of the chordae and valves itself) are indeed strongly associated with MR in dialysis patients. However, they may be secondary to stretching of the annulus, rather than primarily responsible for it. Most authors have not found a correlation with secondary hyperparathyroidism, which causes ectopic calcification in a different localization and pattern. Moreover, calcifications are also very frequent in non-uremic patients with MR. *Valvular calcifications* are reported in 10–40% of HD patients and are more strongly related to disturbed calcium–phosphate metabolism.

Cardiac dilatation, in particular increased left atrial dimensions, is more prominent in patients with MR. Fernandez-Reyes et al. (1995) observed that atrial dilatation preceded *de novo* appearance of regurgitation and calcification. In an analysis of non-renal patients with dilated cardiomyopathy, Boltwood (1983) found a strikingly larger atrial volume and mitral area in patients with MR than in those without MR, while there was no clinical difference between the two groups. He pointed out that the posterolateral annulus is contiguous with the posterior wall of the left atrium which has sparse connective tissue and is therefore more apt to be stretched by enlargement of the atrium. He therefore suggested a 'regurgitation threshold' which, once passed, leads to a vicious circle: 'MR begets MR'.

This consideration is particularly relevant for dialysis patients, who are continuously threatened by (intermittent) overhydration. Volume increase will first stretch the most compliant compartment of the heart, which is the atrium. We have shown that MR and tricuspid regurgitation (TR) can disappear with ultrafiltration: in a group of 21 HD patients, with cardiac dilatation MR (1–4 degree) disappeared in 13 and improved to 1st degree in the remainder. TR 1–4 degree disappeared in 14 and improved to 1st degree in 4 after a mean weight loss of 5.4 kg (Table 8.3).

Tricuspid regurgitation

Tricuspid regurgitation (TR) is most often secondary to mitral or aortic insufficiency. In dialysis patients it is seen together with and proportional to the severity of MR. In our series no case of TR was seen without MR, while three patients had second degree MR without TR. In another series of 32 less overhydrated patients, ten had MR but no TR was detected.

These results leave no doubt that overhydration causing atrial dilatation is the most important cause of MR and TR in dialysis patients. While being a part of the 'dialysis cardiomyopathy' syndrome, their reversibility with appropriate treatment forms one more argument against a 'uremic' cause.

Table 8.3 Regression of mitral (MR) and tricuspid (TR) regurgitation

	Number of patients with					
	MR	TR	MAP	CTi	MA	LVs
Before UF	20	18	126	0.57	23	25
After UF	7	4	95	0.47	19	21

Mean values of 21 patients with mitral (MR) and tricuspid (TR) regurgitation. After intensified UF these improved in all and disappeared completely in 14 of them. This was accompanied by a striking decrease in mean arterial pressure (MAP, in mmHg) cardiothoracic index (CTi) and mitral annular (MA) and systolic left ventricular (LVs) diameters. Diameters are indexed per m^2 body surface area. All changes were highly significant. Data from Cirit et al. 1998.

Aortic valve disease

Aortic stenosis may occasionally be associated with long term dialysis treatment, but regression has not been reported. Both aortic calcifications and valvular disease are closely related to elevated Ca × P product and to a lesser degree to hyperparathyroidism. Aortic valve calcifications are frequent in dialysis patients and often associated with calcifications of mitral valves and annulus. Mild aortic stenosis has been detected in 10% of dialysis patients. Progression of aortic stenosis leading to complaints is unpredictable, but may be very rapid. Once it is discovered, repeated echographic follow-up is indispensable. It should be considered that low BP and decreased systolic function may lead to underestimation of its severity on echocardiographic investigation. When in doubt, invasive procedures are necessary.

Aortic regurgitation is rare. Moderate regurgitation was found in 6% of a selected patient series. Exceptionally severe regurgitation has been reported, caused by a calcification from the atrioventricular septum perforating the left coronary leaflet. Before the advent of echocardiography, rather frequent diastolic murmurs have been attributed to aortic regurgitation, but these may in reality have been from pericardial origin.

Treatment of severe aortic valve disease consists of valve replacement with a metallic prothesis, because a bioprosthetic valve may rapidly become calcified. Like with other surgical interventions in dialysis patients, one should not be conservative.

Pulmonary valve regurgitation

This is sometimes manifested by a diastolic decrescendo murmur, and is not uncommon in dialysis patients. Doppler examination showed pulmo-

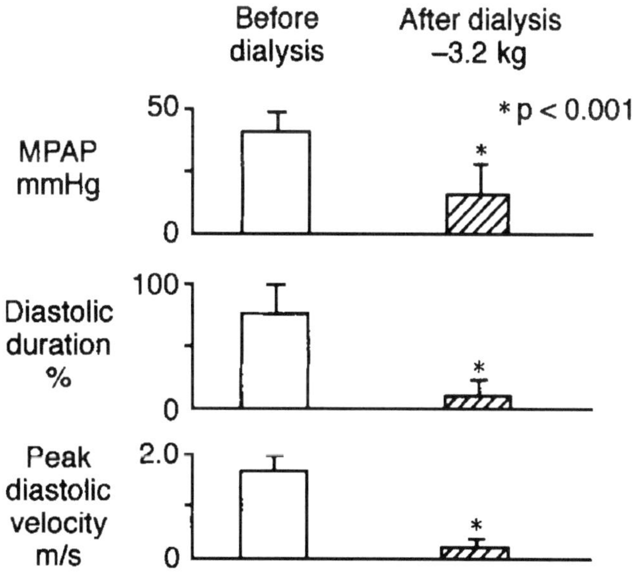

Figure 8.6 Mean pulmonary artery pressure (MPAP), duration and velocity of pulmonary diastolic regurgitant flow in nine patients with functional pulmonary regurgitation before and after UF dialysis (from Perez 1985, with permission).

nary regurgitation in about 10% of the patient population in one study (Perez et al. 1985). In all of them ultrafiltration of ±3.2 L caused a marked decrease in pulmonary artery pressure and almost eliminated the regurgitation (Figure 8.6). Thus, like mitral and tricuspid regurgitation, this form is also functional and caused by volume overload. It reflects reversible pulmonary hypertension.

5 DILATED CARDIOMYOPATHY OF END-STAGE RENAL DISEASE

Semantical discussion

The term 'uremic cardiomyopathy' is often used to indicate a variety of cardiac structural and functional abnormalities. However, it is not well defined and there are reasons to avoid the word 'uremic' and use the non-committal term 'dilated cardiomyopathy of end-stage renal disease' instead.

Discussions whether or not the qualification 'uremic' is justified have been going on for 25 years. Yet, stressing the possible harm of the uremic toxin may divert the attention from preventable factors as will be discussed below. Not surprisingly, dilated cardiomyopathy is particularly frequent in patients with diabetes mellitus (due to the multiplicity of risk factors). Usually the term 'cardiomyopathy' is applied to patients with grossly dilated heart and disturbed systolic and diastolic functions, and in whom cardiac failure persists despite achievement of the assumed dry weight. When HD patients and patients with primary hypertensive heart disease are compared, no differences in diastolic disturbances are found, arguing against specific uremic damage. Most authors therefore agree that the problem is semantic. (Hung et al. 1980).

Mechanisms

Many abnormalities in dialysis patients may contribute to cardiac damage, as they are exposed to known as well as less clearly defined risk factors, both before and during the dialysis treatment. As a result, the prevalence of organic heart abnormalities is high. These can lead to various forms of functional failure.

Hypertension and left ventricular hypertrophy

These cause not only an increase in muscle mass but also structural alterations such as increased interstitial tissue and decreased capillary density (Amann et al. 1995). Functional disturbances like decreased ejection fraction may result from increased wall stress if hypertrophy does not keep pace with the increased volume load. Systolic functions may normalize when the pressure load is relieved, but diastolic disturbances will persist much longer.

Volume overload

The chronic, continuous or intermittent hypervolemia of dialysis patients causes dilated (eccentric) hypertrophy. According to the La Place Law, volume increments need a proportional increase in wall thickness in order to normalize wall stress. In compensated volume overload, peak *systolic* wall stress and ejection fractions are normal, but end diastolic pressure and wall stresses remain elevated. Eventually, increases in end-diastolic and end-systolic volume will mark the occurrence of cardiac damage. In a group of HD patients with low ejection fraction and dilated heart, reduction by ultrafiltration caused improvement of systolic function but only after some time (Hung et al. 1980). In another series a marked improvement of severe heart failure (increase of ejection fraction from a mean of 27% to 56%) was observed within two weeks after transplantation (Burt et al. 1989). Such rapid improvement strongly suggests that 'volume' rather than toxic factors were involved.

Anemia

This has been shown to cause left ventricular hypertrophy (see Chapter 10) probably by inducing a high-output state. In addition low hemoglobin levels may (by hypoxia?) directly cause cardiac damage.

Coronary artery disease

This is highly prevalent in HD patients as can be expected from the frequency of hypertension and diabetes mellitus among them. It contributes significantly to cardiac damage.

Hyperparathyroidism

This elevated Ca × P product in the blood regularly complicate dialysis treatment. Metastatic calcifications in arteries and the periarticular region as well as (less conspicuous) elevated calcium content of various organs, including the heart, are the result. Indeed several authors have found a relationship between hyperparathyroidism and cardiac damage, and improvements after parathyroidectomy have been reported.

Other toxic factors

Animal experiments have clearly shown that renal failure causes fibrosis in the myocardial interstitium independent of hypertension and other abovementioned factors (Amann et al. 1995). Similar observations were made in patients. In addition increased muscle mass and alterations of the myocardial isomyosin pattern was noticed. Several metabolic alterations have been detected in HD patients who may be involved in myocardial and vascular damage. Among them are increased homocystein levels, increased oxidative stress and endothelial dysfunction. The relative importance of these observations has yet to be established.

Treatment

Whatever structural alterations are present, fluid retention plays a contributory and critical role. When a normal heart can fail with volume overload, a diseased heart will suffer even more, and good volume control is more urgent than ever. Remarkable improvements in clinical and echocardiographic disturbances can be achieved by judicious ultrafiltration in such patients (Table 8.4), anginal complaints can be relieved, appetite can improve, etc. It is very difficult to judge how much of the condition of such a patient is due to volume overload per se. Particularly when gross cardiac dilatation and systolic dysfunction are present, patience and perseverance by the dialysis team are required, because adaptation and 'remodeling' of the stretched heart muscle take time to complete. But as every patient is different, treatment is necessarily empirical, guided by close clinical observation. The case history described below illustrates these points.

For nearly 200 years, *digitalis* was the only available cardiac drug. However, its therapeutic margin is narrow and indiscriminate application

Table 8.4 Clinincal improvement by slow UF in cardiomyopathy

	kg	MAP	CTi	LA	EF (%)
Before UF	78	103	0.61	41	30
After UF	59	95	0.49	32	40

Results obtained by repeated, prolonged ultrafiltration (UF) during 1–3 weeks in 5 patients with cardiomyopathy. Mean values. kg = body weight in kilograms; MAP mean arterial pressure (mmHg); CTi cardiothoracic index on chest X-ray; LA left atrial diameter; EF ejection fraction. (Unpublished observations from Ege University Dialysis Centre, Izmir, Turkey)

has raised concern as to whether the numbers of patients profiting from its use exceed those suffering from toxicity. Moreover, the advent of other drugs has limited the indications for digitalis both as an antiarrhythmic and as a 'cardiotonic'. Recent studies, however, have confirmed its beneficial inotropic action in selected patients (i.e. chronic heart failure on optimal diuretic and CEI treatment).

In *renal patients,* digitoxin (not digoxin) should be used. this being metabolized in a non-renal pathway. In *hemodialysis patients,* however, the rapid changes in serum K level (on which digitalis action as well as toxicity are critically dependent) make it impossible to achieve effective digitalization. In addition, as volume expansion is the main pathogenic factor, there will be hardly any need for digitalis, and its benefit in dialysis patients has never been demonstrated. Taken together, there is no place for digitalis, with the possible exception for arrhythmias that cannot be controlled by other means.

With *converting enzyme inhibitors,* apart from their benefit in certain forms of hypertension and left ventricular hypertrophy, there is no information available about their possible adjuvant role of CEI in dilated cardiomyopathy.

Case history

A 16-year-old girl had been admitted to another hospital 2.5 years previously with terminal renal failure (reflux nephropathy) and blood pressure of 240/140. Hemodialysis (twice a week for three hours, later three times for 3.5 hours) was started and BP decreased to 165/110. However, her condition gradually deteriorated and ultrafiltration was not possible because of hypotension.

On admission she was extremely emaciated, hardly able to walk and anorexic. Body weight was 28 kg, length 1.50 m. Her belly was tense and distended with ascites, but there was no peripheral edema. BP was 100/70 mmHg, chest X-ray showed cardiomegaly (CTI 0.72) and on the echocardiogram 3–4 the degree mitral and tricuspid regurgitation was present, but no pericardial effusion. Systolic and diastolic functions were greatly impaired (ejection fraction 17%). In short, a classic example of 'uremic' cardiomyopathy. Treatment consisted of daily dialysis alternated with ultrafiltration sessions, which often caused severe complaints and hypotension. However, while her body weight initially dropped to 23 kg, general condition gradually improved and a tremendous appetite started. After two months the left atrial diameter was reduced and regurgitations decreased, but cardiomegaly and left ventricular functions showed little improvement. By continuing the same treatment strategy, however, all abnormalities gradually disappeared and left ventricular mass decreased from 300 to 150 g. By the fifth month CTI was 0.47, body weight had risen to 33 kg and she had grown 5 cm. One year later a successful kidney transplantation was performed. Some details are shown in Figure 8.7.

Summary

- Some dilatation of left atrium and ventricle are frequent in dialysis patients, suggesting slight, unrecognized volume retention.

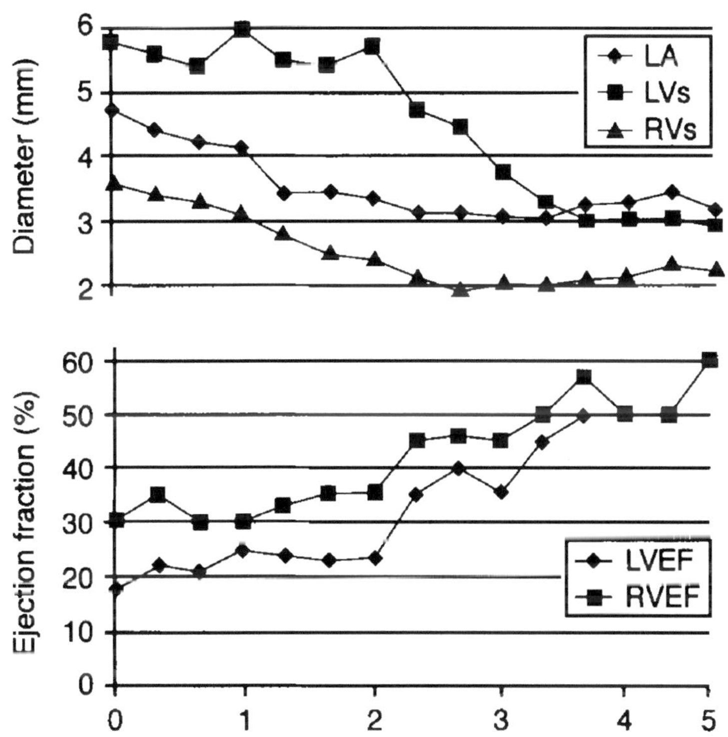

Figure 8.7 Echocardiographic changes during ultrafiltration treatment in a 16-year-old girl with severe dilated cardiomyopathy. Note that during the first 2 months, left atrial (LA) and right ventricular systolic diameters (RVs) decreased, while left ventricular dilation (LV systolic diameter) only improved later. Functions of the left and right ventricle, as evidenced by their ejection fractions (LVEF and RVEF respectively) also recovered only after 2 months (adapted from Töz 1998).

- Hypervolemia probably is an independent risk factor.
- Left ventricular hypertrophy (LVH) is frequent, often progressive and associated with increased risk.
- LVH is due to both pressure (hypertension) and volume overload. The latter is caused by fluid retention, anemia and A-V shunts.
- Regression of the LVH has been reported after treatment of anemia and after blood pressure decrease by volume correction, but seldom after antihypertensive drugs alone.
- Pulmonary congestion and edema are frequent, but preventable by good volume control. While they may occur with a normal heart, cardiac damage aggravates their development. In particular diastolic dysfunction, related to LVH, lowers the threshold.
- On the other hand, pulmonary lymph drainage adapts to longstanding subclinical congestion, allowing higher pulmonary artery pressures without edema.
- Valvular regurgitation, in particular of the mitral, tricuspid and pulmonary valves, is not infrequent (but often unrecognized) in dialysis patients. They are most often functional (caused by cardiac dilatation) and therefore can be corrected by ultrafiltration treatment.
- 'Uremic' cardiomyopathy is ill defined, and the term suggests that toxic factors are responsible. Because this may discourage necessary intervention we propose instead: 'Dilated cardiomyopathy of ESRD'.
- Next to all other damaging factors, longstanding hypervolemia is the most important cause of left ventricular damage, resulting in low ejection fraction and ultimately a decrease in blood pressure.
- With few exceptions, there is no place for digitalis in hemodialysis patients.
- Marked improvement of dilated cardiomyopathy can often be achieved by judicious ultrafiltration. One extreme example of such a patient is given.

Bibliography

Amann K, Neususs R, Ritz E et al. Changes in vascular architecture, independent of blood pressure in experimental uremia. Am J Hypert. 1995;8:409–17.

Boltwood CM, Tei C, Wong M et al. Quantitative echocardiography of the mitral complex in dilated cardiomyopathy: the mechanism of functional mitral regurgitation. Circulation. 1983;68:498–508.

Bonow O, Udelson E. Left ventricular diastolic dysfuncions as a cause of congestive heart failure. Ann Intern Medicine. 1992;117:502–10.

Bryg JR, Gordon PR, Migdal SD. Doppler detected tricuspid, mitral or aortic regurgitation in end-stage renal disease. Am J Cardiol. 1989;63:750–3.

Buoncristiani U, Fagugli RM, Pinciaroli MR et al. Reversal of left ventricular hypertrophy in uremic patients treated with daily hemodialysis. In: Clinical hypertension in nephrology. Karger, Basel ed. 1996:152–6.

Burt RK, Gupta S, Suki WN et al. Reversal of left ventricular dysfunction after transplantation. Annals Int Med. 1989;111:635–40.

Canella G, Paoletti E, Barocci S et al. Angiotensin converting enzyme gene polymorphism and reversibility of uremic left ventricular hypertrophy following long-term antihypertensive therapy. Kidney Int. 1998;54:618–26.

Cirit M, Özkahya M, Soydas C et al. Disappearance of mitral and tricuspid regurgitation in haemodialysis patients after ultrafiltration. Nephrol Dial Transplant. 1998;13:389–92.

Fernanez-Reyes MJ, Bajo MA, Robels P et al. Mitral annular calcification in CAPD patients with low degree of hyperparathyroidism. Nephrol Dial Transplant. 1995;10:2090–5.

Foley RN, Parfrey Ps, Harnett JD et al. The prognostic importance of left ventricular geometry in uremic cardiomyopathy. J Am Soc Nephrol. 1995;5:2024–31.

Golf S, Lunde P, Abrahamsen M et al. Effect of hydration state on cardiac function in patients on chronic haemodialysis. Br Heart J. 1983;49:183–6.

Grossman W, Jones D, McLaurin P. Wall stress and patterns of hypertrophy in the human left ventricle. J Clin Invest. 1975;56:56–64.

Harnett JD, Foley RN, Kent GM et al. Congestive heart failure in dialysis patients. Prevalence, incidence, prognosis and risk factors. Kidney Int. 1995;47:884–90.

Hung J, Harris PJ, Uren RF et al. Uremic cardiomyopathy effect of hemodialysis on left ventricular function. New Eng J Med. 1980;302:547–51.

Katz AM. Cardiomyopathy of overload. New Eng J Med. 1990;322:100–10.

London GM, Fabiani F. Marchais J. Uremic cardiomyopathy: an inadequate left ventricular hypertrophy. Kidney Int. 1987;31:973–80.

London GM, Marchais SJ, Guerin AP et al. Cardiac hypertrophy and arterial alteration in end-stage renal disease. Haemodynamic factors. Kidney Int. 1993;43(Suppl. 4): 42–9.

Michel P. Aortic stenosis in chronic renal failure patients treated by dialysis. Nephrol Dial Transplant. 1998;13(Suppl. 4)44–8.

Özkahya M, Ok E, Cirit M et al. Regression of left ventricular hypertrophy in haemodialysis patients by ultrafiltration and reduced salt intake without antihypertensive drugs. Nephrol Dial Transplant. 1998;13:1489–93.

Perez JE, Smith CA, Meltzer VN. Pulmonary valve insufficiency: a common cause of transient diastolic murmurs in renal failure. Ann Int Med. 1985;103:497–502.

Raine AEG. Acquired aortic stenosis in dialysis patients. Nephron. 1994;68:159–68.

Ribeiro S, Ramos A, Brandao A et al. Cardiac valve calcifications in haemodialysis patients: role of calcium-phosphate metabolism. Nephrol Dial Transplant. 1998;13:2037–40.

Rostand SG, Drücke TB. Parathyroid hormone, vitamin D and cardiovascular disease in renal failure. Kidney Int. 1999;56:383–92.

Silberberg JS, Barre PE, Prichard SS et al. Impact left ventricular hypertrophy on survival in end-stage renal disease. Kidney Int. 1989;36:286–90.

Szidon JP. Pathophysiology of the congested lung. Cardiol Clin. 1989;7:39.

Töz H, Özerkan F, Unsal A et al. Dilated uremic cardiomyopathy in a dialysis patient cured by persistent ultrafiltration. Am J Kidney Dis. 1998;32:664–8.

Wallin CB, Jacobson SH, Leksell LG. Subclinical pulmonary oedema and intermittent haemodialysis. Nephrol Dial Transplant. 1996;11:2269–75.

9 Vascular disease

Functional and histopathological abnormalities are present at all levels of the vascular system in dialysis patients. Even in the capillaries of the nails, Maastricht investigators have described abnormalities, but the clinical consequences have not yet been elucidated. We will therefore confine the discussion to the veins and the large arteries.

1 THE VENOUS SYSTEM

The veins of dialysis patients show morphological changes consisting of increased thickening of the media by smooth muscle cell proliferation (Kooman et al. 1995). This is reflected by a decrease in compliance of the venous system that has been mentioned in Chapter 6 and may sensitize the patient to acute changes in blood volume. Interestingly, these abnormalities were only found in patients with hypertension. This makes it unlikely that they are caused by some 'uremic' toxic factor. An attractive hypothesis is that they are the result of (intermittent) long-standing volume expansion.

2 THE ARTERIAL SYSTEM

The function of the aorta and large arteries is not only to deliver blood to the tissues; they also damp the pulsations by their elastic property (compliance $= \Delta/P/\Delta V$). Two distinct pathological changes are seen in dialysis patients: a general stiffening with dilatation and loss of compliance, which some authors call *arteriosclerosis*, and which interferes with this second function; and *atherosclerosis*, which is more localized in nature and can obstruct blood supply by plaque formation.

Arteriosclerosis

This is primarily a degeneration of the media of the large arteries. It consists of diffuse fibro-elastic intima thickening, increased medial collagen with secondary fibrosis, calcification and dilatation. The mechanisms underlying this increased arterial stiffness are not known, but it seems that overhydration, independently from blood pressure changes, directly alters mechanical properties of the arterial wall.

Calcifications of the large and medium-sized arteries, seen in elderly patients and in diabetics, are particularly frequent in dialysis patients. While often present at the start of treatment, they progress with time and are nearly always seen in long-term survivors (more than 15 years on dialysis). Disturbed bone metabolism with elevated Ca × P product in the blood is probably the main etiological factor.

The result of the stiffening process is loss of the cushioning or 'Windkessel' function, which normally keeps about 50% of the stroke volume and delivers this 'stored energy' gradually to the tissues during diastole. This decreased compliance causes an *increase in systolic* and a *decrease in diastolic* blood pressure. Another consequence of decreased elasticity is that the *pulse wave velocity* increases. This forward travelling (incident) pressure wave, generated by the heart, causes a reflected (echo) wave from the end of the arterial tree upstream. The incident and reflected wave combine to yield the pressure wave. Normally the two components do not co-incide, but with increased wave velocity they come in phase, causing a further increase in amplitude of the pulse wave (Figure 9.1).

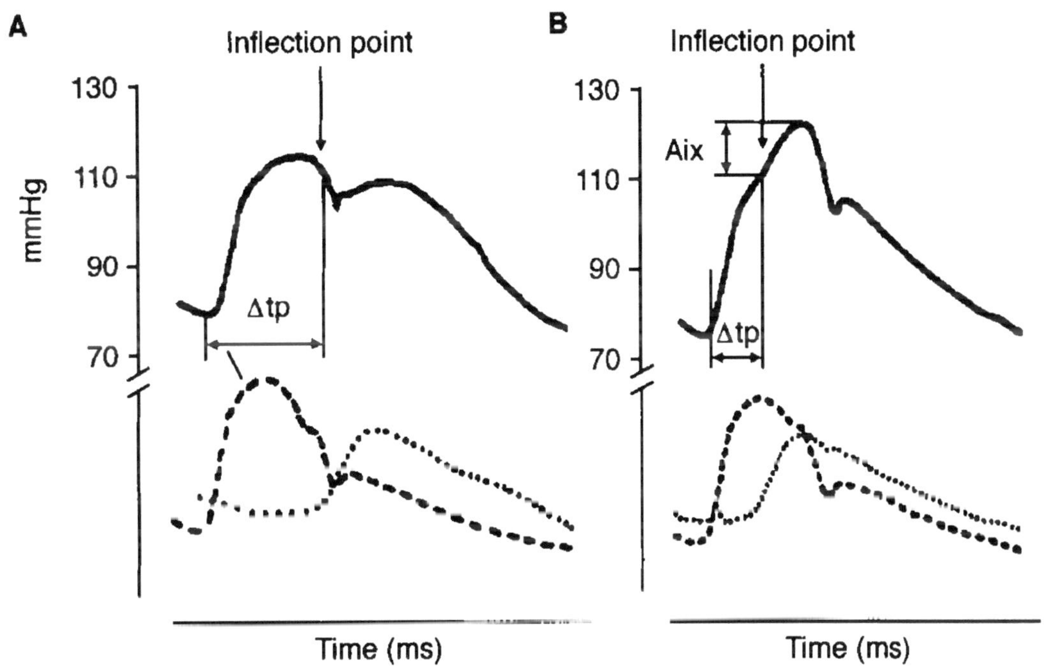

Figure 9.1 A. Recorded ——, incident – – and reflected · · · · · pulse waves in the aorta of a normal person. The sum of the incident and reflected waves yield the recorded wave. B. The same recording from a sclerotic aorta Because the travel time of the reflected wave is faster, it reaches the aorta earlier and the interval with the incident wave (Δtp) is shortened resulting in an amplified pulse wave (Aix = amplification index). From London et al. 1994, with permission.

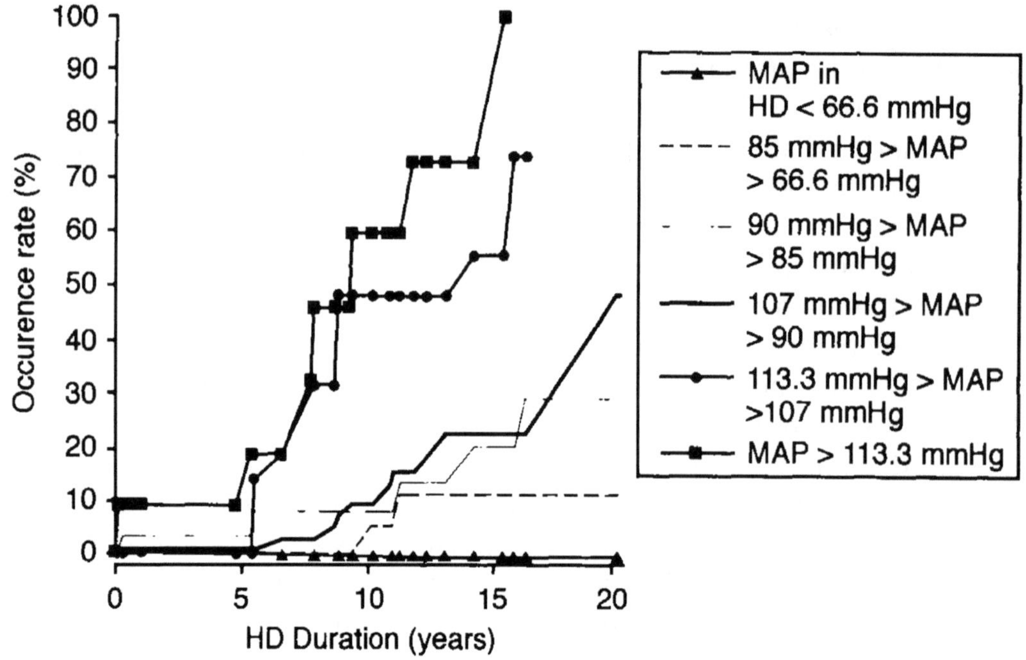

Figure 9.2 Occurrence rate of first atherosclerotic event as a function of MAP in 326 low risk HD patients. From Charra et al. 1994 (Ch. 4), with permission.

The decrease in cushion function as well as the increase in wave velocity together increase the afterload and myocardial oxygen consumption. At the same time mean diastolic pressure is decreased. This will tend to impair coronary blood supply, in the very patients whose oxygen demand is increased. It is not surprising that (as shown in Figure 8.3) a correlation exists between pulse wave velocity and left ventricular hypertrophy. These considerations also explain why systolic BP is a stronger risk factor than diastolic pressure in dialysis patients.

Treatment

Because pulse wave velocity is very much dependent on the existing blood pressure, lowering the blood pressure will decrease this velocity. It has been shown that ACE inhibitors, in addition to their blood-pressure-lowering effect, decrease the pulse wave reflections (London et al. 1996). Beta-blockers increase wave reflections as a result of bradycardia and therefore lower aortic systolic pressure less than that measured in the brachial artery.

Atherosclerosis

The second very important pathological process, which is much increased in dialysis patients, is atheroslerosis, basically an intimal, focal event.

Atherosclerosis is responsible for the very frequent complications like cerebral accidents, aortic aneurysms and coronary thrombosis.

Earlier suggestions that dialysis treatment accelerates atherogenesis have not been confirmed. Rather the multiplicity of risk factors already present before dialysis treatment – and which unfortunately persist during dialysis – provide sufficient explanation for the high numbers of vascular events.

The following risk factors for atherosclerosis can be identified:

Hypertension

Increase in blood pressure is among the most important risk factors for atherosclerosis in the general population. Although it is not strictly proven this probably applies to the dialysis patients as well, as suggested by the experience of the Tassin investigators (Figure 9.2).

Hypervolemia

Besides promoting hypertension, the increased volume may be for a small part localized in the arterial compartment and be responsible for the increase in diameter and wall stress that has been found in large arteries of dialysis patients.

Cigarette smoking

Just as is the case for other risk factors the effect of this important risk factor is even worse in patients with renal disease. Although a strikingly increased mortality in smoking dialysis patients was demonstrated long ago, this issue attracted little attention in the dialysis world.

Lipid abnormalities

Patients with end-stage renal disease have a number of abnormalities in blood lipids, the most common being increased triglyceride levels. However, hypertriglyceridemia is only weakly associated with coronary artery disease. While *serum cholesterol* is often decreased (Figure 9.3), more complex lipid disturbances have been described, notably elevated apolipoprotein-A levels. Decreased HDL cholesterol is known to decrease the anti-atherogenic defense mechanisms.

More important may be finding of increased plasma *homocystein* levels in patients with renal failure, these being only modestly reduced by dialysis. Homocystein has recently been identified as an independent risk factor for coronary artery disease. As will be discussed in Chapter 12 *chronic infections* may also play a role. While all these abnormalities may contribute to

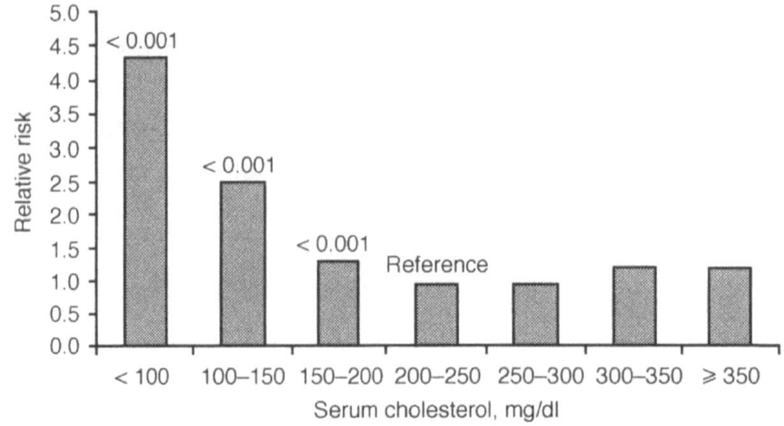

Figure 9.3 Relative risk of death by serum cholesterol among 12 000 hemodialysis patients. Low cholesterol, being a marker of poor general condition is associated with the highest risk! There is a striking parallel with the U curve of hypertension risk. From Coresh et al. 1998, with permission.

atherogenesis in dialysis patients, definite proof of this contention has yet to be provided and at present they seem to be less important than the other mechanisms mentioned above.

Recently, *oxidative stress* has been implicated in the pathogenesis of heart disease, in particular coronary sclerosis in non-renal patients. Several studies have shown a strong association between intake of the antioxidant vitamin E and decreased cardiac risk. Because uremia is a 'pro-oxidant state' it is biologically plausible that oxidative stress also contributes to cardiovascular disease in dialysis patients. However, these results may not be generalizable to this population. Such an association has not been established and prospective studies are lacking (Rigatto and Singal 1999).

Diabetes Mellitus

Diabetic patients suffer from increased atherosclerosis and its consequences, and consequently diabetes constitutes a serious risk factor. When they are on dialysis, all the risk factors related to that treatment not only add up, but actually potentiate this already elevated risk.

Calcium phosphate metabolism

Vascular calcifications are abundant among dialysis patients and increase with the duration of dialysis treatment. They are mainly caused by the abnormal calcium, phosphate and bone metabolism, and to some degree are nearly inevitable. Calcifications are strongly related to the product of calcium and phosphate in the blood. Also when secondary to atheroma they may exacerbate arterial disease, but separate analysis is difficult and this issue is still being debated.

Uremic factors

Atherosclerotic plaques are not static obstructive lesions but dynamic structures that are susceptible to rupture and coronary thrombosis. As emphasized by Ritz and co-workers the evolution of these plaques in uremic patients differs from that in the non-uremic state. It is characterized by more pronounced thickening of intima and media of the coronary vessels, stronger calcifications and striking infiltration of the plaques by activated macrophages. In short, plaques in uremic patients give rise to early thrombosis and seem to be more malignant (Schwarz et al. 1999). This may partly explain the discrepancy between angiographic stenosis and coronary events, as myocardial infarction can be caused by thrombosis without significant stenosis.

3 CORONARY ARTERY DISEASE

Coronary artery disease is extremely frequent in dialysis patients and therefore merits a more detailed discussion. Due to the atypical symptomatology in this condition it is also much underdiagnosed. Systematic screening with angiography in patients who were candidates for transplantation has revealed significant coronary stenosis varying from 24% in relatively young non-diabetic patients up to 85% in elderly diabetics. These figures are many times higher than in a non-renal population. Many patients developing symptomatic coronary artery disease during dialysis treatment had been diagnosed with coronary sclerosis before, and no correlation is present between the duration of dialysis treatment and the occurrence of coronary events. The incidence of fatal coronary events reported varies between 3 and 45 times that observed in the general population, depending on the age and countries, but the incidence and age of onset of first myocardial infarction is similar in predialysis and dialysis patients.

Symptoms

For reasons that are not completely clear there is a poor relationship between the classic symptoms of angina pectoris and angiographical abnormalities. Some studies have shown that one-third of patients with anginal complaints have open coronary arteries while this symptom was absent in nearly half of those with proven stenosis. Dyspnea may be a sign of coronary heart disease but due to the frequent co-existence of pulmonary congestion this symptom is non-specific. Because classic symptoms are often absent, the doctor should be on the alert for other complaints such as abdominal pain, vegetative symptoms and any discomfort related to exercise or time of the day.

Risk factors

Apart from being related to atherogenesis in general, coronary disease may be particularly favored by the following:

Hypertension

Elevated arterial pressure is associated with increased work load and oxygen demand of the left ventricle and therefore likely to aggravate myocardial ischemia.

Hypervolemia

By increasing cardiac preload, volume expansion increases left ventricular filling pressure, the more so when its wall is hypertrophied. According to one study, diastolic filling pressure in dialysis patients is on the average twice that of healthy people. When dilatation is present, wall stress increases proportionally more.

Left ventricular hypertrophy (LVH)

LVH, by decreasing left ventricular compliance, causes a vertical displacement of the diastolic pressure–volume relationship (Figure 8.5). This shift of the relation is exaggerated during ischemia. As coronary perfusion depends on the pressure gradient between aortic and left ventricular pressure during diastole, it is clear that hypervolemia *per se* may increase myocardial ischemia. In addition it promotes interstitial fibrosis in the non-infarcted myocardium. LVH is associated with decreased capillary density and thus compromises the needs of the increased muscle mass.

Anemia

This has a strong but reversible negative effect on coronary reserve. The combination of decreased oxygen supply and the increased workload of hypercirculation can explain this. The attending *tachycardia* is probably the most unfavorable factor since it shortens the diastolic period during which coronary perfusion almost exclusively takes place.

Factors provoking angina

Increased oxygen demand

Hypertension and hypercirculation due to volume retention will increase the likelihood of complaints. Elevated wall stress (see Chapter 8) increases oxygen requirement. Arteriovenous shunts have a similar effect.

Decreased oxygen supply

While ultrafiltration will reduce symptoms related to hypervolemia, intermittent excessive falls in blood pressure are obviously more dangerous in the presence of coronary diseases. Patients with frequent dialysis hypotension episodes have a higher incidence of coronary accidents.

Diagnostic procedures

Angiography

Because atherosclerotic coronary disease, even when asymptomatic, is associated with markedly increased allograft failure and mortality, transplantation candidates suspected of coronary artery disease are usually subjected to coronary angiography. An angiogram is also needed when revascularization is being considered.

Electrocardiogram

Many patients, in particular those with diabetes, have electrocardiographic abnormalities at rest, often related to left ventricular hypertrophy. Failure to attain a sufficient heart rate during exercise makes interpretation difficult.

Scintigraphy

Thallium imaging after dypiridamol has been advocated as a non-invasive method to identify patients with increased risk of cardiovascular outcome. However, reports on their predictive value are conflicting.

Echocardiography

Two-dimensional echocardiography during dobutamine infusion (dobutamine stress test) has been reported to predict death and coronary complications with a high sensitivity and specificity.

Treatment

Risk factor intervention

Correction of anemia This is probably the most effective measure to be taken for symptomatic relief. Prevention of *hypervolemia* and *hypertension* will not only improve symptoms but also prevent progression of the disease. As remarked by Wizemann (1996) "Underdiagnosis, undertreatment, and frequently ignorance have contributed to perpetuate arterial hypertension in the dialysis patient as the single most important clinical problem in nephrological every day routine. For obvious reasons this is particularly true in the hypertensive dialysis patients with coronary artery disease." Dialysis sessions of long duration will allow to titrate the patient to reach an adequate target weight and avoid dialysis-associated hypotension. Theoretically peritoneal dialysis would be the preferred treatment.

Drugs

Organic nitrates are time-honored because they achieve sustantial reduction in left ventricular preload without reflex tachycardia. However, diastolic disfunction requires individual dose adjustment. Medication which causes tachycardia or increased myocardial oxygen demand, such as cathecolamines, should be avoided. If hypertension appears to be renin dependent, angiotensin-lowering drugs are to be preferred. Beta-blockers have the additional advantage of slowing down the heart rate but on the other hand, increase pulse wave reflections. As discussed in Chapter 8 there is hardly any place for digitalis treatment in dialysis patients.

Invasive treatment

Percutaneous transluminal angioplasty appears to be accompanied by many acute and chronic complications and a high recurrence rate in patients with renal failure. This may be related to the instability of the plaques. Consequently it is not generally recommended. In contrast surgical coronary bypass grafting, while having a somewhat higher mortality than in patients with normal renal function, may be remarkably successful in symptomatic dialysis patients, provided they are well prepared for the operation.

4 OTHER COMPLICATIONS CAUSED BY ATHEROSCLEROSIS

Cerebral infarcts and hemorrhage

There is no doubt that cerebral accidents are an important cause of morbidity and mortality in dialysis patients. Due to lack of reliable registration of causes of death the relative contribution of this complication is unknown. For instance, the recent exhaustive report of the US Kidney Foundation on cardiovascular disease did not include cerebrovascular disease and peripheral vascular disease. A recent review from France reported that 10% of occlusive events were cerebral infarctions. There may be large regional differences. Hypertension is of course a strong risk factor for hemorrhage.

Aortic aneurysm and large artery obstruction

In a Japanese study, aortic aneurysm was found to be a main cause of death in dialysis patients, but this probably does not apply to other regions. Nevertheless the paucity of data on this subject precludes a sound judgement. The same applies to occlusive disease of the lower limbs. Particularly in diabetics, but also in other long-surviving dialysis patients, obstruction of ileac and femoral arteries may cause disabling and deadly complications. Statistical data are lacking.

5 SUDDEN DEATH

Sudden death, which is nearly always of cardiovascular origin, is frequent in dialysis patients. There is, however, a paucity of data as to the underlying causes. This is understandable: the patient often dies at home and autopsy is seldom requested. One Japanese publication reported that dissecting aortic aneurysm was the most frequent cause of sudden death, followed by cerebral hemorrhage and infarction, acute subdural hematoma and acute myocardial infarction.

Arrhythmias and cardiac arrest are an important cause of death in dialysis patients. Left ventricular hypertrophy is associated with a high incidence of arrhythmias, particularly when interstitial fibrosis is pronounced. The sudden changes in electrolyte levels in the blood during dialysis much favor their occurrence.. They are particularly frequent after a long interdialytic period as happens in the weekends.

Summary

- Arteriosclerosis (stiffness of the large arteries) is very frequent. It increases the workload of the heart both by loss of cushion function and by increasing pulse wave reflections.
- Blood pressure reduction decreases pulse wave reflections, as do converting enzyme inhibitors.
- Many well-known risk factors for *atherosclerosis* are present in dialysis patients, and consequently vascular events are many times more frequent than in the general population.
- While 'uremia' probably does not accelerate atherosclerosis it makes atheromatous plaques unstable and thus promotes early thrombosis.
- Lipid abnormalities and increased homocystein levels contribute to atherosclerosis, but treatment of more easily preventable factors like smoking, hypertension and anemia should be given priority, because the risk factors potentiate each other.

- Symptoms of coronary artery disease are often atypical and one should be on the alert to detect them.
- Surgical coronary bypass grafting has proved to be more successful than transluminal angioplasty, and dialysis treatment is no contraindication for surgery.
- It is not known what proportion of sudden death is due to cerebral accidents, myocardial infarction, arrhythmias or rupture of aortic aneurysm.

Bibliography

Avram MM, Blaustein DA. Causes, risks and therapy of hyperlipidemia in chronic dialysis patients. Sem Dialysis. 1997;5:267–271.

Coresh J, Longenecker JC, Milles ER et al. Epidemiology of cardiovascular risk factors in chronic renal disease. J Am Soc Nephrol. 1998;9:24–30.

Kooman JP, Daemen M, Wijnen R et al. Morphological changes of the venous system in uremic patients. Nephron. 1995;69:454–8.

De Lemos, Hills LD. Diagnosis and management of coronary artery disease in patients with end-stage renal desease on hemodialysis. J Am Soc Nephrol. 1996;7:2044–54.

London GM. Increased arterial stiffness in end-stage renal failure: why is it of interest to the clinical nephrologist? Nephrol Dial Transplant. 1994;9:1709–12.

London GM, Pannier B Vicant E et al. Antihypertensive effects and arterial haemodynamic alterations during angiotensin converting enzyme inhibition. J Hypertens. 1996;14:1139–46.

Orth SR, Stöckmann A, Conradt C and Ritz E. Smoking as a risk factor for end-stage renal failure in men with primary renal disease. Kidney Int. 1998;54:926–31.

Rigatto C, Singal PK. Oxydative stress in uremia. Sem Dialysis. 1999;12:91–6.

Robinson K, Gupta K, Dennis V et al. Hyperhomocysteinemia confers an independent increased risk of aterosclerosis in end-stage renal disease and is closely linked to plasma folate and pyrdioxine concentration. Circulation. 1996;94:2743–48.

Schwarz U, Amann K, Ritz E. Why are coronary plaques more malignant in the uremic patient? Nephrol Dial Transplant. 1999;14:224–5.

Takeda K, Harada A, Okuda D. Sudden death in dialysis patients. Nephrol Dial Transplant. 1997;12:952–5.

Vincenti F, Amend WJ, Abele J et al. The role of hypertension in hemodialysis-associated atherosclerosis. Am J Med. 1980;68:363–9.

Wizemann V. Points to remember when dialysing patients with coronary disease. Nephr Dial Transplant. 1996;11:236–8.

10

Effusions in serous cavities

In situations where the extracellular volume is increased, the excess fluid will accumulate in any part of the body where the tissues have sufficient compliance to accept it. Therefore not only the subcutaneous space (edema) but also the spaces between serous membranes which are 'empty' in normal man can be filled with fluid. Special lymph drainage systems exist in the three main compartments – pericardial, pleural and peritoneal cavities – ensuring a negative pressure in normal conditions.

Overhydration is not the only cause of fluid accumulation, which may have a completely different pathogenesis in each of them.

1 PLEURAL EFFUSION

Several causes of pleural effusions should be distinguished.

Overhydration

Pleural effusions of small amounts are very frequent in fluid-overloaded dialysis patients. They are seen in conjunction with cardiac dilatation and pulmonary congestion and may be predominantly unilateral as fluid accumulates preferentially at the side the patient is lying on. Sometimes interlobular accumulation may give a tumor-like appearance. They rapidly subside with appropriate ultrafiltration.

Uremic effusions

In some dialysis patients, serosanguinous or even hemorrhagic effusions can be found in the absence of overhydration. Pleural biopsy reveals signs of chronic 'fibrinous pleuritis'. They may be rather resistant to treatment with thoracentesis and intensified dialysis, and are suspected to be related to some viral infection. Indeed there is an analogy with uremic pericarditis (see below) with which they often coincide.

Other causes

Tuberculosis is frequent in dialysis patients and is particularly difficult to diagnose as classic symptoms may be mild or absent. Tuberculous pleuritis may be present without lung lesions on chest X-ray.

All other causes of pleural effusion like cancer, embolism, bacterial infection (empyema) etc. may of course also be present in dialysis patients. During peritoneal dialysis (CAPD) a *diaphragmatic leak* can give rise to massive, usually right-sided hydrothorax.

Treatment

When effusions do not rapidly subside with adequate ultrafiltration, pleural puncture is indicated for diagnostic purposes. If the effusion is large, withdrawal of fluid may accelerate recovery.

2 PERICARDITIS

Pericarditis is one of the most important complications of end stage renal disease and was once a sign of imminent death. Before the dialysis era, it was present in more than half of the patients dying from uremia. It was found in a high proportion of patients starting dialysis treatment, but its frequency has diminished with earlier start of this treatment. Still it is reported in 5–15%. While it usually disappears with frequent dialysis, it continues to be a problem, also during chronic dialysis. The following types can be distinguished.

Infectious

Infectious pericarditis may be primary, due to tuberculosis or due to secondary infection with pyogenic bacteria. This is reason to perform a pericardial punction when in any doubt.

Hypervolemia

Small to moderate hypervolemia-associated effusions can be detected by echocardiography, a method which is sensitive enough to detect amounts as small as 20 ml. They are asymptomatic and disappear with adequate ultrafiltration.

Uremic pericarditis

This is the classic type which disappears with intense dialysis treatment. However, it may re-appear after months or years in patients considered to be adequately dialyzed. Therefore some authors distinguish a separate entity: 'Dialysis-associated pericarditis'. This appears *de novo* in patients who are feeling well on chronic dialysis treatment and cannot be distinguished on clinical or biochemical grounds from those without pericarditis. It has therefore been attributed to a viral infection, which, however, has not been identified. Its frequency is estimated around 8%, while the incidence is less (2–4%) in CAPD patients. This observation would suggest some toxic (uremic) origin, perhaps 'middle molecules' which are better removed by the latter treatment. This form of pericarditis is often triggered by some 'stressful event' like an operation or infection. In one large series, no difference in response to treatment was found between pericarditis before ('uremic') and during maintenance dialysis, casting doubts on the distinction between both forms. We will therefore discuss them together.

Symptoms of uremic or dialysis-associated pericarditis are quite characteristic, but they are by no means definitive.

- *Pain*, in the pericardium, sometimes irradiating to the left shoulder is present in 70% of the cases. It may be related to the position of the body.
- *Fever* and moderate *leucocytosis* is seen in 60% of the patients.
- *A friction rub* may be very loud or absent and, contrary to general belief, is not related to the amount of fluid. It may come and go, thus requiring regular auscultation.
- *The pericardial fluid* is always bloody.
- In 50% of the patients some *pleuritis* is also present.
- ST abnormalities on the ECG, which are characteristic of other forms of pericarditis, are nearly always absent! Depending on the amount of fluid, low voltage may be present.

Treatment

Because of the probability that some uremic toxin is involved, the frequency of dialysis sessions should be increased. As the pericardial fluid is always bloody, it is logical to minimize heparinization. Regional heparinization does not usually ensure normal clotting time in the patient and is not advised any more. The effectiveness of none of these measures has been documented. Because overhydration and hypertension seem also to contribute, better ultrafiltration should be part of this strategy. In this way 60% of pericarditis disappears within two weeks. The remaining patients take longer to recover and are sometimes very resistant. Treatment with prednisone and NSAID has been tried, but their effectiveness has not been proven.

Factors predicting failure of conservative treatment are high temperature on admission, elevated white blood cell count ($>15\,000/\text{mm}^3$), large effusions (both anterior and posterior by echocardiography), low blood pressure and signs of hemodynamic instability (de Pace et al. 1984).

Cardiac tamponade is a serious, potentially dangerous complication that calls for early intervention. It is more likely to occur early in the course of the disease. As it may happen suddenly, close clinical supervision is needed. It has been shown that collapse of the right atrium during right ventricular systole on echocardiography is an early sign, followed by ventricular collapse during diastole, which precedes a decline in systemic arterial blood pressure (Singh et al. 1984). Immediate relief can be obtained by pericardiocenthesis, which is performed by introducing an 18-gauge needle by the subxiphoid approach under electrocardiographic control, followed by a catheter with multiple side holes. Many physicians are reluctant to perform this procedure for fear of puncturing a coronary vessel. However, when the effusion is large, the risk is low in experienced hands and most probably the numbers of patients dying because the intervention was postponed are far greater than those who succumbed from complications of the puncture.

When the effusion is large and persistent, emptying by puncture may relieve symptoms and fever, but recurrence is frequent. More permanent improvement can be obtained by surgical fenestration by subxiphoid pericardiostomy under local anesthesia. As the effect may be limited by the presence of localized effusions, particularly at the posterial wall, pericardectomy under general anesthesia is the best solution. This will also prevent development of *constrictive pericarditis.* However, contrary to expectation this complication has rarely, if ever, been described as a sequel of dialysis-pericarditis.

3 ASCITES

Dialysis patients are more prone to developing ascites-associated diseases than are healthy people. The following causes can be distinguished:

Cirrhosis of the liver

Because of the frequent occurrence of infectious hepatitis and decreased immune competence, ascites and cirrhosis develop more frequently and at an earlier stage. The diagnosis should not be difficult.

Infectious peritonitis

Spontaneous *bacterial peritonitis* is fairly common in HD patients, probably favored by pre-existing fluid accumulation. Since it may be relatively asymptomatic, early diagnosis by puncture and aggressive antibiotic treatment are mandatory. *Tuberculous peritonitis* is also more frequent in dialysis patients. The diagnosis may be difficult, and large amounts of ascitic fluid (with sedimentation) should be examined to increase the chance of detecting acid-fast bacilli (for details see Franz and Hörl 1997). Malignant tumors may cause ascites by obstructing veins and lymph nodes as well as by carcinomatosis peritonea. The important thing is to differentiate them from the following entities:

Fluid overload

With the extreme degrees of fluid overload which sometimes happen in ESDR and insufficiently treated HD patients, the fluid may accumulate in the abdominal, as well in other cavities. It usually subsides with appropriate UF treatment. However, ascites sometimes persists when other fluid collections disappear. Some authors (Hammond and Takiyyuddin 1994) consider this as a specific entity: 'Nephrogenic or dialysis-associated ascites'.

Nephrogenic ascites: fact or fiction?

The reported incidence of this mysterious condition varies between 0.7 and 26%. The diagnosis is made *per exclusionem*: when no other causes can be found and the ascites are not cured by ultrafiltration, 'nephrogenic ascites' is assumed to be present. The prognosis of these patients is very poor and half of them die within a year, usually showing cachexia. Drastic treatment methods like peritonea-venous shunts have been proposed. Peritoneal dialysis will (almost by definition!) relieve the ascites and improve the condition. One report showed the beneficial effect of treatment with converting enzyme inhibitors. It is of note that rapid cure was reported after successful transplantation: out of 24 patients 22 had complete resolution of the ascites within 2–6 weeks. This observation argues for a disturbed fluid balance as the primary cause. Yet additional factors like disturbed lymphatic drainage may explain why certain patients are particularly sensitive. While it is hard to deny the existence of a new entity, the strong variation of its reported frequency suggests that at least in some cases the presumption that it is resistant to ultrafiltration may not be correct. Personally I have not encountered a single patient whose ascites could not be relieved by persistent UF. However, these patients constitute a *special entity*: they have severe overall cardiac damage, most have low blood pressure (although previously they often had severe hypertension). Right-sided heart failure predominates over pulmonary congestion, and venous pressure is elevated. Edema may or may not be evident, but liver congestion can be found both on physical examination and by echography. As a result, mild liver function disturbances are frequent, appetite is minimal and malnutrition is the rule. In short, the condition resembles the old concept of 'cardiac cirrhosis'.

The patient whose cardiac condition was described in the case history in Chapter 8 is a typical example. Besides cardiomegaly and venous congestion, abdominal ultrasonography showed severe ascites with congestion of the hepatic veins and the liver. Liver functions were slightly disturbed (bilirubin 2.7 ml/dl). Upon the strict ultrafiltration strategy applied, congestion and anorexia rapidly disappeared and bilirubin normalized. It took about six weeks for the ascites to disappear completely, while the cardiac abnormalities needed much more time to recover (see Figure 8.7).

Summary

- Pleural effusions are often due to overhydration and may give unusual pictures on the chest X-ray. The possibility of other causes, in particular tuberculosis, should be kept in mind.
- Pericarditis is a symptom of terminal renal failure, but may also occur in seemingly well-dialyzed patients. A viral origin has been suggested in some patients, but proof is lacking.
- Intensified dialysis (and ultrafiltration if possible) usually lead to recovery within two weeks, but effusion may be very resistant. In such cases pericardiectomy may be required.
- Cardiac tamponade is a real danger, particularly in the early phase. Pericardiocentesis should not be postponed out of fear of complications.
- Ascites may have several causes such as overhydration, peritonitis and liver disease.
- There is no conclusive evidence for the existence of 'nephrogenic ascites' as a separate entity. Many of such cases are associated with heart failure (cardiac cirrhosis).

Bibliography

de Pace NL, Nestico PF, Schwartz AB. Predicting success of intensive dialysis in the treatment of uremic pericarditis. Am J Med. 1984;76:38–48.

Franz M, Hörl WH. The patient with end-stage renal failure and ascites. Nephrol Dial Transplant. 1997;12:1070–78.

Hammond TC, Takiyyuddin MA. Nephrogenic ascites: a poorly undestood syndrome. J Am Soc Nephrol. 1994;5:1173–77.

Singh, S, Wamm LS, Schuchard GH et al. Right ventricular and right atrial collapse in patients with cardiac tamponnade. Circulation. 1984;70:966–71.

11

Anemia and the heart

Anemia is an almost universal feature of end-stage renal failure and an important contributor to the complaints of these patients. In addition observational studies have identified anemia as an important independent risk factor for general and cardiovascular mortality in dialysis patients. Anemia is – together with hypertension – a major determinant of myocardial dysfunction, and in one study it appeared to be independently associated with left ventricular dilatation and the development of *de novo* cardiac failure.

1 PATHOPHYSIOLOGY

Causes

Three major causes have been distinguished: 1. *Toxic* effects and *chronic infections* resulting in a shortened half-life of the erythrocytes and inhibition of erythropoiesis; 2. *Iron deficiency* (blood loss in dialyser and by blood sampling for analytic purposes) and decreased 'availability' of iron despite normal ferritin levels; 3. Absence or decrease of *erythropoietin* production. The importance of toxic factors is demonstrated by the fact that in one center (Tassin) where long dialysis (24 hours per week) is practiced, the need for erythropoietin treatment is much less than elsewhere.

Pathophysiological consequences

In order to supply the tissues with sufficient oxygen despite decreased oxygen transport capacity of the blood, a general vasodilatation occurs (autoregulation). This results in an elevated cardiac output and a hyperdynamic circulation, which is supported by an increase in venous return and preload. Some increase in blood and extracellular volume must accompany this process (Gerry et al. 1976). Correlations have been found between the degree of anemia, increase in cardiac output and left ventricular volumes and muscle mass. The chronic high output state contributes importantly to the left ventricular hypertrophy and eventually to heart failure. While anemia seriously increases the symptoms of coronary insufficiency, a direct influence on the development of coronary artery disease has not been documented.

2 TREATMENT

The correction of anemia by any means will reverse the high output state and improve many complaints like fatigue, exercise intolerance, lack of appetite, loss of sexual desire and function. While factors 1 and 2 should not be neglected, lack of erythropoietin is by far the most important. The advent of recombinant erythropoietin (Epo) has revolutionized dialysis treatment.

Erythropoietin (Epo) and mortality

As a low hemoglobin level is one of the main risk factors for cardiovascular outcome, a beneficial effect of improvement of anemia by Epo is to be expected. However, long-term prospective multicenter studies have given controversial results. A large Japanese study showed a tendency to increased risk and myocardial infarction in Epo-treated patients. In contrast, an even larger Italian investigation comprising all dialysis patients in a certain region reported a lower general mortality of 11.1% per year in patients treated with Epo as compared to 15.2% in untreated patients (Locatelli et al. 1999). A similar improvement was noticed for cardiovascular mortality. Surprisingly, however, there was no correlation at all between hematocrit level and cardiovascular mortality, while non-cardiac and, to a lesser extent, cerebrovascular death rates were lower in patients with higher hematocrit levels. The authors consequently suggest a beneficial, pharmacological effect of Epo per se, independent of its effect on hematocrit on the condition of the heart. It should be remarked that in these studies (like in many of those analyzing the impact of dialysis treatment in general) no mention was made of blood pressure and the condition of the heart. It is necessary therefore to discuss in more detail the possible untoward effects of Epo treatment that might confound the beneficial results of anemia correction, in particular its purported hypertensive action.

Erythropoietin hypertension

Most studies dealing with Epo have reported the appearance or worsening of hypertension, which may necessitate interruption of the treatment. This 'Epo hypertension' has the following peculiarities: 1 (Dorhout Mees 1997). Hypertension does not develop in patients with normal renal function; 2. The incidence of hypertension varies markedly between published series. In large multicenter trials, the incidence of hypertension (defined as a rise in blood pressure or an increase in the requirement of antihypertensive drugs) was reported between 26% and 58%, although in one study no change in average blood pressure was seen. Patients with pre-existing hypertension are said to be particularly at risk. Seizures have been reported, but mostly in patients with a history of seizures. In contrast, no rise or even some decrease in blood pressure was described in other papers dealing with smaller numbers of patients. 3. No correlation between rise in blood pressure and the dose of Epo or final hematocrit level was found. However, a rapid rise in hematocrit is said to increase the risk of hypertension. Furthermore, its frequency is highest during the first few months, and may disappear altogether during maintenance treatments with Epo. 4. Finally it is particularly relevant that in trials comparing Epo with placebo, a significant number of patients on placebo also developed hypertension!

Several investigations suggest indirect effects of Epo like stimulation of endothelin production, endothelial proliferation and other actions on the cellular level, but the clinical relevance of these experimental findings is not evident. Clinical studies have failed to show increases in cathecolamines or renin angiotensin levels during Epo treatment regardless of the blood pressure response. Some show a decrease in plasma renin activity. The most striking events during reversal of anemia by Epo (or any other treatment) are an increase in blood viscosity and an increase in peripheral vascular resistance. They happen whether blood pressure rises or not, and are a physiological reversal of the changes caused by anemia. Consequently most authors blame *inadequate adaptation* or failure of autoregulation as the major cause of Epo-induced hypertension. But why do most patients react adequately while some do not?

The most plausible explanation is *inadequate volume control.* Theoretically, an increase in red cell volume would result in an increased blood volume, unless plasma volume decreases in proportion. Thus if no special care is taken to reduce plasma volume, a hypervolemic state will result even if external fluid balance and body weight are kept constant. Investigations where volume changes were measured during Epo administration support these considerations. One study in which no hypertension was observed showed a decrease in plasma and extracellular volume while blood volume did not change. In contrast, another study where blood pressure increased, reported a marked increase in blood volume. Most relevant is the investigation of Anastassiades et al. (1993) who compared the effects of Epo in CAPD patients with predialysis patients. Despite similar increases in hematocrit and red cell volume, blood pressure slightly decreased in the former and increased in the latter. Plasma volume decreased in the CAPD group but not in the predialysis patients, whose blood volume increased markedly (Table 11.1). This difference evidently reflects the better feasibility of volume control in dialysis patients. We collected 17 studies from the literature (comprising 220 patients) in which no hypertension was observed after Epo (Dorhout Mees and Ok 1997). They usually concerned small but well-controlled series of patients in which details like blood volume and echocardiographic results were documented.

Table 11.1 Relation between blood volume and blood pressure of patients treated with erytropoietin

	Changes after Epo	
	Group 1	Group 2
Mean blood pressure	+10	−1 mm
Red cell volume	+571	+560 ml
Plasma volume	−100	−756 ml
Blood volume	+471	−194 ml

A group of ESRD patients (not yet on dialysis) (group 1) and a group of CAPD patients (group 2) showed a similar improvement of hemoglobin levels after Epo treatment, but only group 1 developed hypertension. In that group, plasma volume remained nearly constant, resulting in an increase in blood volume. In contrast, BP did not rise in the patients of group 2. In that group, plasma volume decreased markedly while blood volume showed a small decrease. Data from Anastassiades 1993.

A common denominator in these studies was a decrease in left atrial and ventricular dimensions and no change or decrease in blood volume. In contrast, patients whose blood pressure increased often showed increases in blood volume and no decrease in cardiac volumes. Thus Epo hypertension is probably due to unrecognized increase in blood volume despite unchanged body weight.

Regression of LVH

Anemia is (together with hypertension) an important cause of hypertrophy of the left ventricle. The responsible mechanism is the *hyperdynamic state,* which burdens the heart, in other words increases *volume load.* Several studies have shown that correcting anemia with Epo both improves the function and modifies the structure of the heart. This applies particularly to regression of LVH. However, such improvement has not been observed in patients who become hypertensive -and thus probably hypervolemic. The relative ease and rapidity with which anemia correction decreases LVH strongly support the important role of (subclinical) volume load and increased wall stress in the pathogenesis of LVH. This contrasts with the failure to achieve regression of LVH in the majority of dialysis patients treated with antihypertensive drugs, and forms one more argument for the predominant role of volume in dialysis-related LVH.

Adjuvant therapy

In order to achieve optimal results of Epo treatment *iron supplementation* is nearly always necessary. Because iron absorption by the gut is disturbed, intravenous administration is advised. As remarked in the beginning of this chapter, erythrocyte survival is reduced in patients with renal failure. Increased ATP alterations in phospholipid membrane components and impairment of the pentose–phosphate shunt have been reported. Deficiency of L-carnitine is believed to be a key factor in some of these alterations, which are *not corrected* by Epo treatment. As its metabolism is certainly disturbed in dialysis patients, L-carnitine deficiency has been blamed for a variety of abnormalities without convincing proof. There is some evidence that L-carnitine supplementation may improve response to Epo. However, a consensus group recently concluded that it should only be used as a trial in patients who are resistant to Epo or need very high dosage. It should not be used in the presence of elevated C-reactive protein, very high PTH levels or aluminum toxicity, which are all conditions known to cause or aggravate anemia.

ACE inhibitors and erythropoietin

It is well known that ACE inhibitors may cause anemia. This effect is thought to be mediated by inhibition of Epo production in the native kidneys. However, ACE inhibition also seems to diminish the effect of administered Epo, at least in high dosages. As low-dose ACE inhibitors are only required in the few patients whose hypertension is resistant to volume control, the practical importance of this interesting feature is limited.

3 SHOULD HEMOGLOBIN LEVELS BE COMPLETELY NORMALIZED?

Initially it was a custom only to correct partially anemia with Epo. In 1997, American Guidelines advised a target hemoglobin level of 11–12 gr/dl. This was evidently based on the notion that morbidity caused by anemia increases significantly when hemoglobin levels fall below 10 gr/dl. The high cost of Epo, but also the concern that higher levels might carry unknown risks, probably contributed to this choice. Indeed it was found that normalizing hematocrit increased thrombosis of arteriovenous fistulas. Incidentally the dose of Epo (and costs!) required for complete normalization of hematocrit is more than three times higher than for partial correction. Therefore several prospective trials have been performed which compare the results of partial versus complete correction. Unexpectedly, these large and expensive trials have not solved the problem (Jacobs 1999). In two studies no difference was found with respect to safety and cardiovascular events while quality of life improved significantly. Another compared the effects of treatment in patients with and without LVH, and showed that while normalization of hemoglobin prevented progressive dilatation and LVH in patients with normal left ventricular volume, it failed to induce regression of dilatation and LVH in those with pre-existing dilatation. It was concluded that normalization of hemoglobin should be done early. While this may be good advice, the failure to correct these abnormalities while others, as discussed above, have clearly shown that this is possible, leads to the tentative conclusion that the patients in this trial were not adequately treated with respect to volume control. Most disappointing were the results of the very ambitious American Normal Hematocrit Cardiac Trial which had to be prematurely stopped because of excess mortality in the normal hematocrit group (Besarab et al. 1998). This caused a wide-ranging debate regarding the interpretation and statistical analysis used. Subsequent analysis suggested that factors other than hematocrit itself were responsible for the outcome. In particular, the patients randomized to the normal hematocrit group showed a decline in KT/V values (and volume control?) while KT/V increased in the low hematocrit group. In addition, the entry criteria required these patients to have high cardiac risk. This means that they were particularly sensitive to volume excess. Anyway the results cannot be extrapolated to low-risk patients, and contrast with the previously mentioned Italian study where patients with the highest hematocrit had no change in cardiac death rate, and some improvement in overall death rate. In conclusion, this issue is (and probably will remain) unsolved.

Summary

- Anemia causes hyperdynamic circulation which results in left ventricular hypertrophy and dilatation.
- Anemia has been identified as an independent risk factor for cardiac mortality. In addition anemia increases symptoms of coronary disease and in general compromises the patients' well being.
- The main causes of anemia in dialysis patients are iron deficiency, toxic ('uremic') metabolites, which inhibit erythropoiesis and increase erythrocyte life span and insufficient production of erythropoietin.
- Treatment with recombinant Epo can reverse all the ill effects of anemia. However, the frequent occurrence or worsening of hypertension appears to be a drawback.
- Arguments are presented for the contention that 'erythropoietine hypertension' is a condition caused by unnoticed expansion in the blood volume.
- The issue whether complete normalization of hemoglobin levels has advantages over partial correction of anemia is still being debated.

Bibliography

Anastassiades E, Howard D, Howard J et al. Influence of blood volume on the blood pressure of predialysis and peritoneal dialysis patients treated with erythropoietin. Nephrol Dial Transplant. 1993;8:621–5.

Besarab A, Bolton WK,. Browne JK et al. The effects of normal as compared with low hematocrit values in patients with cardiac disease who are receiving hemodialysis and erythropoetin. New Eng J Med. 1998;339:584–90.

Dorhout Mees EJ, Ok E. Erythropoietin hypertension: fact or fiction? Int J Artificial Organs. 1997;20:415–7.

Foley RN, Parfrey PS, Harnett JD et al. Impact of anemia on cardiomyopathy, morbidity and mortality in ESRD. Am J Kidney Dis. 1996;28:53–61.

Gerry JL, Baird MG, Fortuin NJ. Evaluation of left ventricular function in patients with sicle cell anemia. Am J Med. 1976;60:968–72.

Goldberg N, Laudin AP, Delano B et al. Changes in left ventricular size, wall thickness and function in anemic patients treated with recombinant human erythropoietin. Am Heart J. 1992;124:424–7.

Jacobs C. Normalization of hemoglobin: why not? Nephrol Dial Transplant. 1999;14(Suppl. 2):75–9.

Locatelli F, Cante F, Marcelli D et al. The impact of haematocrit levels and erythropoietin treatment on over-all and cardiovascular mortality and morbidity (Lombardy study). Nephrol Dial Transplant. 1998;13:1642–44.

London G, Zins B, Pauwler B et al. Vascular changes in hemodialysis patients in response to recombinant human erythropoietin. Kidney Int. 1989;36:878–82.

Macdogall JC, Lewis NP, Saunders MJ et al. Long-term cardiorespiratory effects of amelioration of renal anemia by erytropoietin. The Lancet. 1990;335:498–503.

Mann JFE. What are the short-term and long-term consequences of anemia in CRF patients? Workshop report. Nephrol Dial Transplant. 1999;14(Suppl. 2):29–36.

12

Nutritional aspects

1 GENERAL CONSIDERATIONS

The patient with chronic renal failure is very often in a state of *malnutrition*. The insidious uremic intoxication, acidosis and overhydration cause a gradual loss of appetite, energy and exercise. In addition, the traditionally advised low-protein diet, aimed at postponing the uremic state, may aggravate the negative protein balance.

The start of dialysis treatment often marks a striking increase in well being and initiates an anabolic period. Indeed, a gradual increase in 'dry weight' during the first months of treatment can be considered as proof of successful dialysis.

In the early years of hemodialysis, it was common practice to maintain some degree of protein restriction. Since three times a week dialysis and high permeable membranes were applied, more attention was given to protein metabolism. Using nitrogen appearance and other methods it became clear that a diet containing 1 g of protein per kg is desirable to provide optimal nutrition.

Nevertheless many dialysis patients still appear to be undernourished. A recent investigation in Sweden, using the 'subjective global nutritional assessment' method, reported that 51% of hemodialysis patients suffered from mild malnutrition and 13% from severe malnutrition (Bergström et al. 1998). One factor may be the loss of amino acids (in particular branch chained (iso)leucine and valine) during dialysis, but low amino acid levels do not correlate with malnutrition.

2 MALNUTRITION, SERUM ALBUMIN AND MORTALITY

Investigations have revealed a strong association between *malnutrition* (and in particular *low serum albumin* levels), and overall mortality, both in hemodialysis and peritoneal dialysis patients. However, only 5% of mortality is directly due to malnutrition (or 'cachexia').

There are several indirect ways in which malnutrition could predispose to fatal complications. One plausible explanation is that it decreases resistance to infections. Cytosine production by mononuclear cells was found to be suppressed in malnourished dialysis patients. This may contribute to decreased immune response. Elevated CRP levels, a marker of chronic inflammation, is even more strongly associated with mortality than is hypoalbuminemia. Another way in which malnutrition could adversely affect mortality is by deficiency of L-arginine, the precursor of nitric oxide. Insufficient nitric oxide generation, which may also be compromised by elevated ADMA levels, may then contribute to hypertension, cardiac damage and decreased defense against infection. Of course, the chicken-and-egg question appears: low albumin may be *a risk marker* rather than a cause of fatal outcome. The same consideration applies to its relation with *cardiac disease.* There is a parallel with low cholesterol levels which are associated with high mortality in dialysis patients (see Figure 9.3). Moreover it was shown recently that serum albumin levels increased markedly after correction of moderate acidosis. Persistence of moderate acidosis despite 'adequate' dialysis treatment is often a neglected problem in these patients.

3 CHRONIC HEART DISEASE

Heart disease, and congestive heart failure in particular, are well recognized causes of malnutrition. *Hypoalbuminemia* is also strongly associated with (congestive) cardiac failure, ischemic heart disease, left ventricular dilatation and cardiac mortality. An important mechanism is *anorexia,* caused by liver congestion and sometimes digitalis toxicity, while bowel edema may impair absorption. In addition these patients are in a *hypermetabolic state,* due to dyspnea and increased sympathetic activity. It has recently been reported that *cytokines* (tumor necrosis factor, interleukin) are increased in cardiac failure, possibly as a result of tissue hypoperfusion. These cytokines may have multiple harmful effects: increase in protein catabolism, anorexia and decrease in cardiac contractility. They also trigger acute phase response in the liver resulting in elevated CRP levels and increased degradation of albumin. Thus, low albumin levels could be mainly the result of cardiac disease and indirectly of chronic overhydration. On the other hand, unrecognized decrease in lean body mass by malnutrition can mask overhydration and thus contribute to congestive failure, as exemplified in Figure 12.1.

4 INFECTION

Chronic inflammation, to which dialysis patients are more prone than healthy individuals, causes acute phase response with elevated CRP, fibrinogen and lipoprotein-a (Lp[a]) levels, These have all been implicated in the pathogenesis of atherosclerosis and consequently heart disease. These rather complicated (and not yet completely elucidated) interrelationships are illustrated in Figure 12.2.

Finally in severe overhydration, albumin levels are lowered by dilution. In CAPD patients, serum albumin levels were found to be inversely related

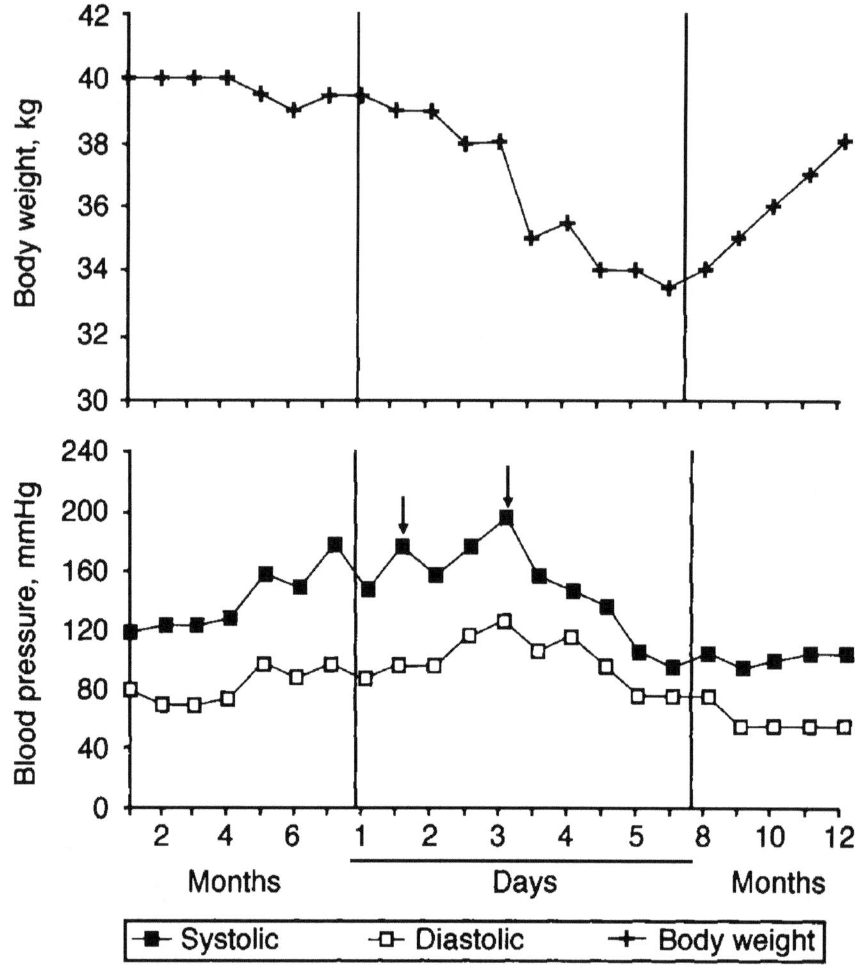

Figure 12.1 Example of a patient who became undernourished, unrecognized because of concomitant fluid retention. This caused hypertension and finally pulmonary edema. After correction by ultrafiltration (note change of time scale) she gained 'real weight' without BP rise.

to extracellular fluid excess. In such patients removal of excess fluid by ultrafiltration may raise albumin blood levels up to 10%.

5 CONCLUSION

Malnutrition and low serum albumin levels are *risk markers* rather than directly involved in mortal complications. Treatment should be directed towards the underlying cause, which most of the time is fluid overload and sometimes unrecognized infection. It is clear that infusion of albumin will be dangerous as it can precipitate heart failure. There is rarely an indication to administer the much advertised amino-acid preparations. A protein-rich meal like beef or yogurt is tastier and has the same effect.

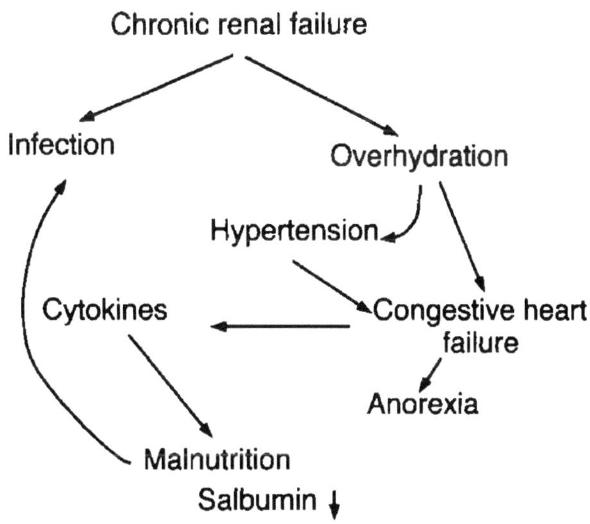

Figure 12.2 Factors contributing to malnutrition in patients with renal failure. Scheme simplified from Bergström et al. 1998.

Summary

- Malnutrition is frequent in dialysis patients and often goes undetected.
- Low serum albumin, which is considered a marker of malnutrition, is independently correlated with overall and cardiac mortality.
- Overhydration and (subclinical) congestive heart failure are well-known causes of anorexia and malnutrition.
- Chronic infections cause acute phase proteins, which are often increased in dialysis patients and thus may contribute indirectly to malnutrition and heart disease.
- Treatment of malnutrition should be directed towards the underlying causes. There is no place for albumin infusions or amino acid administration.

Bibliography

Bergström J, Lindholm B. Malnutrition, cardiac disease, and mortality: an integrated point of view. Am J Kidney Dis. 1998,32:834–41.

Borah MF, Schoenfeld PY, Sargent JA et al. Nitrogen balance during intermittent dialysis therapy of uremia. Kidney Int. 1978;14:491–500.

Foley RN, Parfrey PS, Harnett JD et al. Hypoalbuminemia, cardiac morbidity and mortality in end-stage renal disease. J Am Soc Nephrol. 1996;7:728–36.

Jones CH, Smye SW, Newstead CG et al. Extracellular volume determined by bio-electric impedance and serum albumin in CAPD patients. Nephrol Dial Transplant. 1998;13:393–7.

Ritz E, Vallance P, Nowicki M. The effect of malnutrition on cardiovascular mortality in dialysis patients: is L-arginine the answer? Nephrol Dial Transplant. 1994;9:129–130.

13
Peritoneal dialysis

Continuous ambulatory peritoneal dialysis (CAPD) was introduced in the 1970s and rapidly gained popularity as an alternative mode of dialysis treatment for end-stage renal disease. At present around 30% of ESDR patients are receiving this method of treatment and several scientific journals are exclusively devoted to peritoneal dialysis. There are two reasons why only one chapter of this book is concerned with this subject. The first and most important is that the basic pathophysiological principles involved in cardiovascular complications are the same in hemodialysis and peritoneal dialysis and have been extensively discussed in the previous chapters. The second is that there are very few systematic data available on the most important issue, hemodynamics and volume control, in patients treated with CAPD.

1 CARDIOVASCULAR COMPLICATIONS AND RISK FACTORS

Cardiovascular events and death are as common in CAPD as in HD patients In European series, CV death ranges from 27% to 56% for CAPD and from 25% to 44% for HD. In the USA it fluctuates around 45% for both techniques. These facts are somewhat surprising in view of the theoretical advantages of CAPD over HD, which will be discussed below. A possible explanation for the absence of better outcome may be a different 'case-mix'. Because age and diabetes mellitus are the most important CV risk factors, the inclusion of more older and diabetic subjects in a given patient population would unfavorably affect overall and CV mortality. On the other hand most risk factors are already present during advanced renal failure and much damage has been done before the start of dialysis treatment (Table 13.1). Early start of this treatment while there is still significant residual renal function has always been a general strategy in many CAPD centers. This should give the opportunity for early intervention and prevention. However, CAPD treatment in itself may produce side-effects like obesity and hyperlipidemia that adversely influence CV disease.

As has been pointed out by Lameire (1996), there is a striking change in risk factors with time on dialysis. While some improvement was seen in left ventricular hypertrophy and hypertension in patients who were treated by CAPD for 2–3 years, this is not sustained and at the end of five years

Table 13.1 CV risk factors (%) at the beginning of CAPD treatment in one center (Gent, Belgium)

	Non-diabetic ($n = 201$)	Diabetic ($n = 52$)
BP > 140/90	51	86
Antihypertensive therapy	55	92
Cardiac disease	34	71
CT index > 0.5	58	77

both risk factors were found with the same prevalence as at the start of treatment. These data suggest that there is a continuous negative impact of CAPD treatment per se on the CV status of these patients. The same applies to their state of nutrition. A recent study from the UK (Davies 1998) reported gradual decrease in arm circumference as well as in plasma albumin levels after two years, while many patients died after a period of progressive debilitation. As in hemodialysis treatment there are differences in outcome between centres and countries. Thus the available incomplete evidence suggests that CAPD, in the way it is currently practiced, provides no better CV prognosis than does HD.

2 HEMODYNAMIC AND CARDIAC STATUS

Hypertension

According to the US Renal Data System, 65% of non-diabetic and 87% of diabetic patients on CAPD had inadequate BP control. These figures are at least as bad as, if not worse than, for HD patients. Several studies reported initial improvement – even better than with HD – during the first years of CAPD treatment but at the end of five years the number of antihypertensive drugs used increased in parallel with decreased BP control. An Italian multicenter analysis revealed that hypertension was prevalent in 88% of the patients, in half of them moderate to severe. Of those treated with antihypertensive drugs, 79% remained hypertensive. A recent prospective study from the Netherlands reported mean blood pressure values of 142/85 three months after starting CAPD treatment, despite the fact that 66% of the patients were on antihypertensive medication. In that study mortality was significantly related to systolic blood pressure. There is little doubt that, just as in HD, hypervolemia is also the main cause of hypertension in CAPD patients. Less information is available on other factors like sympathetic activity and circulating BP-raising metabolites in CAPD patients. Sustained, unexplained hypotension is seen in ±5% of CAPD patients. Isolated observations suggest that some patients on CAPD have low BP and hypercirculation with relaxation of peripheral arterioles, but relevant data are lacking.

Cardiac dilatation and failure

Cardiothoracic index (chest X-ray) as well as echographically determined LVH improved (just like hypertension) to start with but deteriorates after some years of CAPD (Lameire 1996).

Figure 13.1 shows a high prevalence of left atrial dilatation and LVH in a group of normotensive CAPD patients. The same investigators noticed an increase of LVH from 52% to 76% of their patients with a parallel increase in cardiovascular mortality. Similarly a high prevalence of left ventricular systolic and diastolic functional disturbances together with LV dilatation and cardiac decompensation was noticed in CAPD patients who did not survive.

The few available studies on this subject suggest that CAPD patients are *constantly overhydrated*, even if compared to HD patients. This is evidenced by the demonstration of a high pulmonary artery pressure, elevated c GMP levels, and by a remarkable reduction of 'dry' body weight when transferred to HD or after transplantation. Some reports show a high proportion (30%) of edema and other symptoms of congestion.

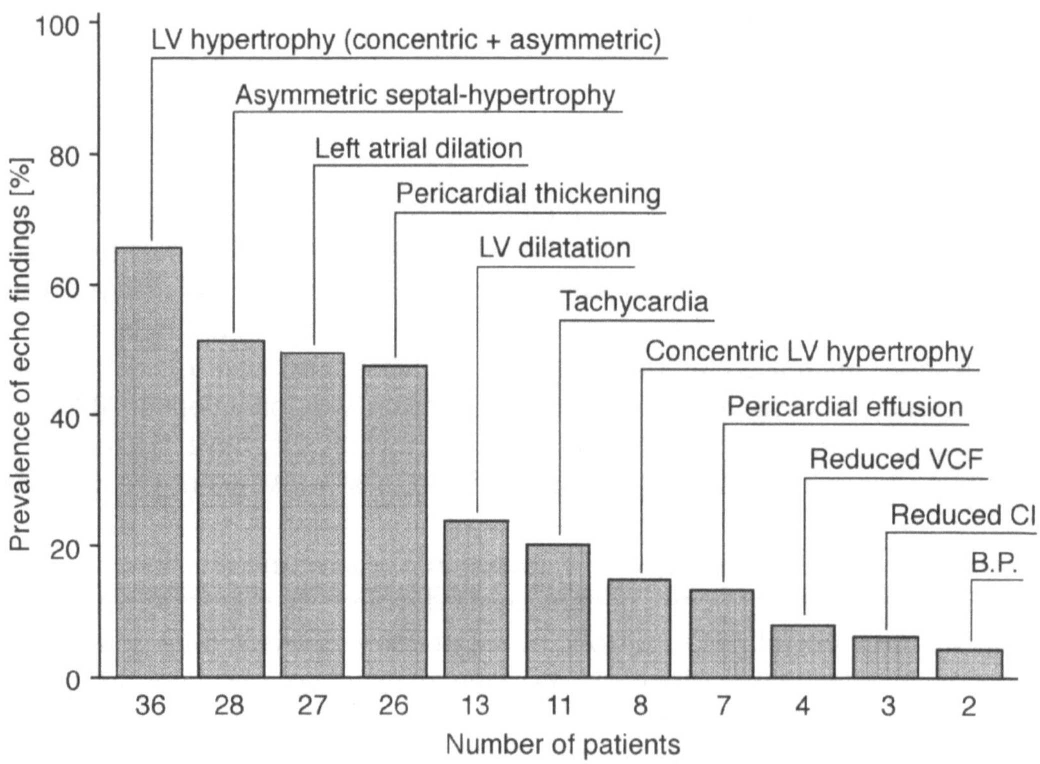

Figure 13.1 Prevalence of pathologic structural and functional echocardiographic findings in 55 patients receiving CAPD (from Hüting et al. 1990, with permission).

Coronary sclerosis

Generally accepted risk factors for atherosclerosis such as hypertension, diabetes mellitus and lipid disturbances are frequent among CAPD patients. Some of these, in particular the lipoprotein metabolism, may be actually worsened by the treatment. Low serum albumin levels are present in all patients due to peritoneal losses. The considerable glucose loads are responsible for the fact that CAPD patients have a more atherogenic lipoprotein profile. In particular higher cholesterol and lower HDL cholesterol and apoA/apoB ratio are reported. The prevalence of coronary heart disease has not been studied carefully in CAPD patients but most probably it is at least as high as in HD patients.

Arrhythmias

Although acute electrolyte changes which occur in HD patients are absent, Holter monitoring shows a high frequency of atrial and ventricular premature beats. They are probably a reflection of left ventricular hypertrophy or underlying ischemic heart disease.

3 TREATMENT OF OVERHYDRATION IN CAPD PATIENTS

Withdrawal of excess salt and water during CAPD treatment is as urgent as it is in HD treatment. This is achieved by creating an *osmotic gradient* between dialysis solution and the patient's body fluids. Glucose, being the cheapest 'natural' osmotic agent, is therefore added to the solution in concentrations varying between 1.5% and 4.25%, which assure an osmotic difference of 70 to 210 m mol/L in excess of the normal blood osmolality of 280 m mol/L. In this way large amounts of EC fluid can be removed. However, due to the fact that the peritoneal membrane is less permeable for charged solutes (ions, such as Na Cl^-), this *osmotic ultrafiltration* attracts relatively more water than NaCl. In other words, the ultrafiltrate is relatively hyponatremic as compared with plasma. This phenomenon is called *sodium sieving* and has important consequences. The net reduction in ECV is less than suggested by the removed volume because the hyponatremic ultrafiltration causes an increase in serum Na concentration that results in increased water drinking. This phenomenon is more pronounced in patients with low membrane permeability (see below) and is enhanced by short dwell-times, as applied in automated PD. The insufficient removal of NaCl probably contributes to volume retention and hypertension. The fluid removal by hyperosmotic (high glucose) dialysate is also unpredictable and has to be adapted individually. Several factors influence this process, the most important one being the condition of the peritoneum.

In addition to drainage problems related to the position of the peritoneal catheter, the main cause of the variability of fluid removal is difference in glucose absorption from the fluid in the peritoneal cavity. The reason is variability in the transport properties for small molecules of the peritoneal membrane (Figure 13.2). The more permeable the membrane, the better urea and other products diffuse from the body, but also more glucose is lost from the dialysis fluid to the body, decreasing the osmotic gradient. Thus what is good for clearing toxic products is bad for removing excess fluid. It appears indeed that 'high transporters' have the lowest survival. When the fluid stays too long in the peritoneal cavity, the profit may be lost. In such patients the UF efficiency can be greatly enhanced by more frequent exchanges and short dwelling times (Figure 13.3), but this goes at the cost of the simplicity of the treatment.

Recently the Izmir investigators (Unal et al. submitted) observed that hypertension could be normalized without drugs in 40 out of 47 patients by salt restriction and increased ultrafiltration. MAP decreased from a mean 117 ± 15 to 92 ± 10 mmHg and CTi from 0.48 ± 0.06 to 0.43 ± 0.05 when body weight was reduced by 2.8 kg. However, there was an immediate decrease in residual urine volume from 720 ± 580 to 272 ± 327 ml per day. These results strongly support the above-mentioned contention that hypertension in CAPD patients is mainly due to volume retention, and also support the hypothesis that volume expansion is an important factor in preserving residual renal function.

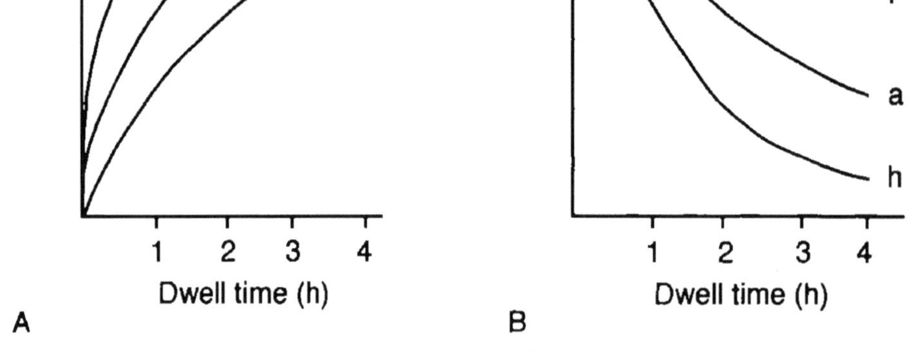

Figure 13.2 Changes in dialysate composition during peritoneal dialysis for patients with *average* (a), *high* (h) and *low* (l) peritoneal permeability. A. *Urea* concentration in dialysate (D) as a fraction of plasma concentration (P). B. *Glucose* concentration (D) as a fraction of initial dialysate concentration (D_0).

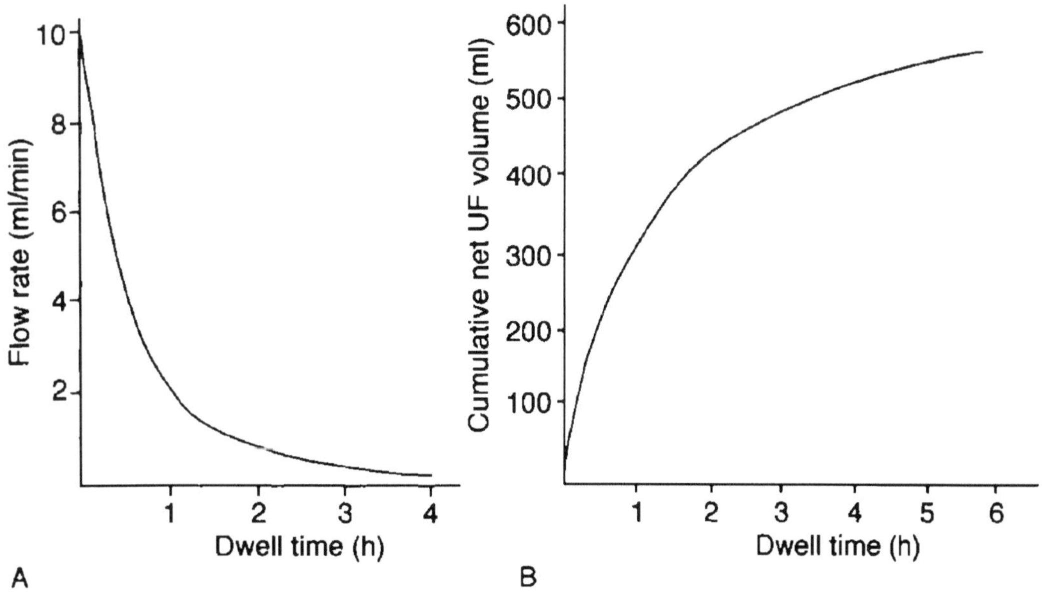

Figure 13.3 Ultrafiltration during hypertonic glucose dialysate. A. Flow rate. B. Cumulative fluid balance (net ultrafiltred amount).

4 WHY DOES CAPD NOT PROVIDE BETTER CV RESULTS?

Fluid removal by peritoneal dialysis is basically much easier than with intermittent hemodialysis because it is done continuously and the problems of dialysis hypotension do not occur. It has been used successfully in the treatment of patients with refractory heart failure and normal kidneys. In patients starting CAPD treatment or transferred from HD, improvement of congestion and better BP control are indeed frequently encountered. However, as indicated before, this improvement is often not sustained. While the reasons for this gradual move from good control can only be suspected, some facts are relevant:

Loss of residual renal function

This is probably the most important reason. Because investigators who originally promoted CAPD realized that the maximal achievable clearance (or in modern terms KT/V) would be only marginally sufficient for adequate removal of urea and other waste products, it became a habit to start CAPD while there was still appreciable renal function. This made it possible to reduce the originally conceived five exchanges to four times a day. It seemed to be an advantage that residual renal function is also preserved for rather a long time during CAPD, while in HD the remaining function of the kidneys is lost much more rapidly. The loss of residual renal function depends on the underlying renal disease, and is more pronounced in glomerular diseases. It has been hypothesized that the decline in renal

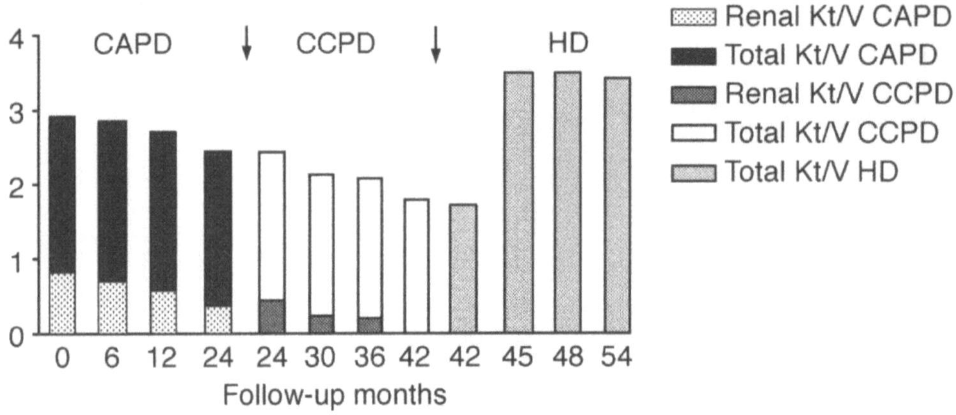

Figure 13.4 Evolution of total and renal weekly KT/V urea in a patient during the successive periods of dialysis treatments. The total KT/V dramatically increased after transfer to HD (from Lameire et al. 1997, with permission).

function during HD is related to the large fluctuations in volume and BP which are common in this form of treatment. They may cause *glomerular vasoconstriction* leading to permanent damage. This theory is supported by the observation that CCPD (nightly cycler peritoneal dialysis) also causes more rapid decline in renal function (Figure 13.4).

An additional and probably more important factor sustaining residual function in CAPD may be that these patients are often continuously volume-expanded (Lameire et al. 1996). If this were true, the obvious advantages of preserved excretory capacities (and probably endocrine functions) must be balanced against the deleterious effects of volume expansion, which need not be repeated here. Thus the desire to achieve a high KT/V comes into direct conflict with the need for good volume control! After what has been said in the previous chapters I need not repeat that volume control should be given the highest priority and if this results in too low a KT/V, (urea removal) dialysis should be intensified.

Lack of volume control

The ease with which fluid can be removed in CAPD together with the residual excretion capacity of the kidneys has led to negligence of salt restriction, while liberal protein intake is encouraged to compensate for the loss of albumin by the peritoneum. Patients were told that the advantage of this mode of treatment was that they could eat and drink as much as they liked. In fact, currently advised salt intake ranges from 130 to 175 m mol/day or even higher!

In view of the above-quoted evidence of overhydration in the majority of CAPD patients, such advice is *not justified.* Apart from the frequent difficulties in withdrawing the necessary amounts of fluid due to outflow problems and loss of ultrafiltration capacity of the peritoneal surface, it seems likely that the possibilities offered by the CAPD technique are often not sufficiently exploited. This may be due to difficulties in determining the 'dry weight' in these patients. Basically the same problem exists during HD, but there the persistence of hypertension during a dialysis session is at least a sign that more UF is necessary. In contrast to HD patients, those on CAPD are not seen several times a week by the dialysis team and much more has to be left to their own responsibility and insight. The latter is heavily dependent on the conviction and convincing power of the physicians and nurses.

Conclusion

Despite theoretical advantages the optimistic expectations of less patient morbidity and mortality on CAPD treatment have not been realized. The reasons for this regrettable development are obvious: difficulties in establishing dry weight and insufficient awareness of latent overhydration, just as in HD, albeit partly for different reasons. To prevent this, dietary salt restriction is the most logical step. If there is sufficient renal function, high-dose loop diuretics may be helpful. But above all the doctors' attention should be diverted from the kidney to heart and circulation; that is, he should become a *metanephrologist.*

Summary

- Cardiovascular complications in CAPD patients are as frequent as in HD patients, but less literature is available on this subject.
- Pathophysiological mechanisms are also the same in CAPD and HD.
- Overhydration and hypertension seem to be less frequent during the first months of treatment, but as time goes by, this advantage is lost.
- Despite the advantage offered by this method to remove excess fluid gradually and thus avoid the problems of 'dialysis hypotension' of HD patients, fluid retention is frequently present.
- Among the reasons for this are gradual loss of residual renal function and increased permeability of the peritoneal membrane for glucose.
- Constant unrecognized volume expansion is probably the main cause of longer preservation of renal function.
- Greater awareness of these problems by both physicians and patients, frequent control visits and more severe salt restriction are among the most logical preventive measures.

Bibliography

Cocchi R, Esposti, Fabri a et al. Prevalence of hypertension in patients on peritoneal dialysis. Nephrol Dial Transplant. 1999;14:1536–40.

Davies SJ, Phillips L, Griffith AM et al. What really happens to people on long-term peritoneal dialysis? Kidney Int. 1998;54:2207–17.

Hüting J, Kramer W, Reitinger J et al. Cardiac structure and function in continuous ambulatory peritoneal dialysis. Am Heart J. 1990;119:344–52.

Jager KJ, Merkus MP, Dekker FW et al. Mortality and technique failure in patients starting chronic peritoneal dialysis. Kidney Int. 1999;55:1476–85.

Lameire N, Vanholder RC, van Loo A et al. Cardiovascular disease in peritoneal dialysis patients. Kidney Int. 1996;50(Suppl. 56):528–36.

Lameire N. the impact of residual renal function on the adequacy of peritoneal dialysis. Nephron. 1997;77:13–28.

Leenen FH, Smith DL. Oreopoulos DG. Changes in left ventricular hypertrophy and function in hypertensive patients started on CAPD. Am Heart J. 1985;101:102–6.

Shetty A, Aftentopoulos IE, Oreopoulos DG. Hypotension on CAPD. Clin Nephrol. 1996;45:390–7.

Tzamaloukas AH, Saddler MC, Murata GH et al. Symptomatic fluid retention in patients on CAPD. J Am Soc Nephrol. 1995;6:198–206.

Unal AJ, Özkahya M, Duman S et al. Normalization of blood pressure by volume control in CAPD patients (submitted 2000).

14

Final considerations and future perspectives

"He who increases knowledge increases sorrow", *Ecclesiastes 1:18*

1 QUALITY OF LIFE

In 1960 Belding Scribner presented the first patients being kept alive by chronic hemodialysis. His message did not generate enthusiasm among nephrologists. Listeners feared not only that the expenses would be prohibitive, but also that most patients would not be able to endure the hardships of this new treatment. Neither of these fears was justified. The high costs turned out to be an incentive for profit-making industry and health care providers. While in the beginning rigid criteria regarding physical, mental and social conditions were considered necessary to select patients fit enough to bear the continuing life restrictions and discomforts of dialysis sessions, today even the oldest and most disabled patients are accepted. Consequently, the condition of the dialysis population has been changed radically. The high proportion of multiple disabilities inevitably decreases the quality of life. It is fortunate therefore that there is a growing interest not only in the assessment but also in improvement of life quality.

Those patients who prefer death to continuing treatment have the lowest quality of life. The steep increase of deaths due to terminating dialysis poses serious ethical problems and urges self-reflection. Should maintenance dialysis never have been started, or did supervening complications make continuation of the treatment meaningless? Insufficient counseling and support during the treatment may also tip the balance in the patients' decision to abandon dialysis. Starting dialysis treatment is only the beginning of a continuing engagement between doctor and patient 'for better and worse'. Unfortunately there is a growing discrepancy between the number of patients and the increasingly scarce time available for patient care. Indeed, the danger that dialysis units turn into 'rinsing factories' is not imaginary. Standardized questionnaires on life quality and checklists registered in data systems (while avoiding 'data overload') would be helpful, but if our profession wants to live up to its traditional standards, *more time for care* (and thus a larger part of the budget) should be made available.

The pathophysiological approach advocated in this book to prevent or improve cardiovascular complications implies that some unpleasant measures have to be imposed in order ultimately to reach a better physical condition and – most probably – a better quality of life. Many patients object to being changed to a stricter regimen, and, particularly if they have been treated before with little obvious harm, the treating staff may also hesitate to force their patients because 'their life is already so difficult'. However, the trouble caused by such measures is often only temporary. The unpalatability of a salt-free diet (the most important condition for improvement) lasts for only a few weeks. As explained in Chapter 6, the discomfort of ultrafiltration also subsides when the goal is reached.

It is sometimes stated that longer or more frequent dialysis sessions are not acceptable for certain populations. However, once transferred to such a regimen, patients usually prefer to continue because they feel much better. It is well known that many patients are not aware of the limitations resulting from a chronic disease until their condition improves. It is the duty of the dialysis team to convince the patient, and 'unwillingness' of the patient should not be used as a pretense for negligence in this regard. Motivating the patients and giving them co-responsibility for their own health are an integral part of dialysis treatment. Non-compliance to treatment is a modifiable risk factor!

The dramatic story of the world's first chronic dialysis patient made a lasting impression on Scribner's approach to the control of blood pressure. It convinced him that 'it requires patience and persistence on the part of the dialysis staff, and willingness to tolerate occasional episodes of cramping and hypotension on the part of the patient' (Scribner 1990). The patient described on page 91 made a similar impression on the author of this book for the treatment of 'uremic cardiomyopathy'.

It is hoped that the interest shown during recent years in the quality of life of our patients will result in increased attention to the individual patient. The finding that home dialysis patients enjoy a better quality of life is probably related to the responsibility given to the patient which is part of this mode of treatment (Kahn 1998). Whatever treatment is applied, it is clear that the doctors responsibility is not limited to 'prescription' of dialysis.

2 EVIDENCE-BASED TREATMENT AND CONTROLLED TRIALS

Evidence has been presented in the preceding pages that it is possible to normalize blood pressure, prevent congestive failure and improve a variety of functional cardiac disturbances in the large majority of dialysis patients. Despite arguments supporting the conclusion that this will lead to decreased morbidity and mortality, definite proof is still lacking. In other words the strict criteria of 'evidence-based medicine' have not been met. In order to do that, controlled trials are needed in which a randomly selected large number of patients have the presumptive beneficial treatment deliberately withheld until their mortality satisfies the statistically required level. It is my conviction that such trials, which have not been carried out for the past 38 years, for practical and ethical reasons will not be performed in the future.

Although it is easy to quote examples where the doctors' 'life-long experience' and honest convictions have meant straying from the correct path, it would not be correct to use the absence of statistical evidence as an argument for continuing a strategy which has not led to expected results. The principles of evidence-based medicine have proven to be beneficial in answering relatively simple questions, like, 'Which drug or operation gives better results?' At present this approach seems to be not applicable to the complicated disabilities of dialysis patients and even brings the temptation of therapeutic nihilism. The next-best solution is to combine application of well-accepted pathophysiological principles, experience in patients without renal disease and some 'uncontrolled', yet impressive results in dialysis patients as a basis for a therapeutic approach. After all, much medical progress in the past has been made without controlled trials.

3 PRACTICAL CONSIDERATIONS

A legitimate question concerns the reason why achievement of some goals, which seem to be within reach, have not been very successful. The answer is that it is indeed difficult to mimic the subtle homeostatic functions of the normal kidneys with the clumsy dialysers (or artificial kidneys, as they were once called) however sophisticated they may be. To realize these goals, much effort and individualized care is necessary and most dialysis doctors simply cannot afford to spend the required time.

The best solution may be to involve the dialysis nurses more in the treatment. They are the ones who have the closest contact with the patients and are in the best position to counsel them. In order to do so, they need a basic pathophysiological understanding of the dialysis treatment. I hope that this book will be helpful in that respect. Once more insight is acquired, more responsibility in the prescription of ultrafiltration, monitoring of blood pressure, interpretation of chest X-ray, etc. could be handled by the dialysis nurse. Very positive results of such an approach were reported from a dialysis centre in Turkey (Sahan et al. 1997). In addition, simple questionnaires on complaints and exercise capacity to monitor signs of over- or underhydration, could be filled by them and used in discussion with the treating physicians. This would serve as a way to increase motivation in the nurses and excite new interest in the sometimes boring routine of the dialysis room. Of course their salaries should be adjusted accordingly.

4 FUTURE PERSPECTIVES

The history of chronic dialysis, only 40 years old, has witnessed many developments that were completely unexpected by medical, psychological and health-policy experts. Dialysis treatment has also appeared not to be immune to fashion. Predicting the future is thus a hazardous, if not a presumptuous endeavor. Accordingly, I will mention only some changes that can be observed in the dialysis world at the time of writing.

Early start of treatment

In the past the start of dialysis treatment used to be postponed until the last moment, not only for economic reasons but also because it was believed that the patient should have experienced serious symptoms, and even felt impending death in order to accept dialysis treatment. Since then, early start of dialysis while there is still residual renal function is increasingly being advocated in order to improve prognosis. This tendency is likely to continue. However, it may be very difficult to prove that this will increase life expectancy and quality of life, and compensate for the extra discomfort and expense. It will come as no surprise to the reader that in my opinion, it is not the removal of toxic products, but better volume control, which should be the main goal. Cardiovascular damage, mainly caused by chronic overhydration, starts indeed long before end-stage renal failure is reached. While treatment of hypertension in the earlier stages of renal disease not only prevents cardiac damage but also retards progression of renal failure, efforts to decrease volume and attempts to lower blood pressure with drugs in advanced stages often result in decreased glomerular filtration rate. Good volume control without dialysis is difficult and is often not attempted for fear of losing residual function. By timely application of salt restriction and loop diuretics, overhydration may be prevented and the heart protected, but at the cost of declining renal function, necessitating dialysis. The result of such an approach may still be an early start of dialysis, but the difference lies in the intention. If dialysis is started without correcting blood pressure and volume overload, the efforts may be in vain.

Co-morbidity

One of the main blessings of dialysis treatment is that it prepares patients for a successful renal transplantation. For a variety of reasons, many patients do not get this opportunity. The increasing acceptance of patients with additional health problems together with the selection of younger and fitter persons for transplantation increases the proportion of co-morbidity in the population that remains on dialysis. However, cardiovascular events have also become the main cause of death in transplanted patients (15 times more than in healthy controls). This development emphasizes once more the need for early intervention. The main cause of co-morbidity is *diabetes mellitus*, which greatly increases the risk of cardiovascular disease, thus potentiating the risk already inherent in chronic renal failure. As overhydration-related hypertension is particularly disastrous in diabetic patients, early intervention is mandatory in this group. As other neurological and ocular complications seriously impair the already compromised quality of life of a dialysis patient, good regulation of diabetes should be given the same attention as adequacy of dialysis. Similar considerations apply to coronary disease and other co-morbid conditions. Defeatism regarding the final outcome often leads to *undertreatment*. It is clear that these developments make it all the more necessary for the dialysis doctor to be an all-round, compassionate physician.

Comeback of clinical research?

Despite the general trend in medical research towards molecular biology, there is no doubt that many questions related to more general pathophysiological disturbances have remained unanswered, particularly regarding blood pressure regulation. Some of them have been mentioned in the preceding chapters. Dialysis treatment constitutes an almost ideal model for investigation of many problems, which cannot be solved in the laboratory. Unfortunately, the nature of chronic dialysis treatment makes it seem a dull routine. Yet every patient presents his own, unique problems. Medicine is only 'routine' for those with a routine mind. I hope that this book will convince the readers that our knowledge is far from complete and that occasions to contribute to it are within the reach of every clinician.

Bibliography

Henderson LW, Thuma RS. Quality assurance in dialysis, 2nd edn. Kluwer Academic Publishers, Dordrecht 1999.

Kahn JH. Co-morbidity: the major challenge for survival and quality of life in end-stage renal disease. Nephrol Dial Transplant. 1998;13(Suppl. 1):76–9.

Kutner NG, Brogan D, Kutner MH. End stage renal disease treatment modality and patients quality of life. Am J Nephrol. 1986;6:396–402.

Liberatti A, Telaro E, Perma A. Evidence-based medicine and its horizons: a useful tool for nephrologists? Nephrol Dial Transplant. 1999;14(Suppl. 3):646–52.

NKF Dialysis quality and clinical practice guidelines. Am J Kidney Dis. 1997;30: (Suppl. 2 and 13).

Sahan F, Ornek H, Gök E et al. Contribution of dialysis nurses to blood pressure and volume control. Turkish National Nephrology Congress. 1997.

Scribner BH. A personalized history of hemodialysis. Am J Kidn Dis. 1990; 16:511–19.